Navigating Organized Urology

Stephen Y. Nakada · Sutchin R. Patel
Editors

Navigating Organized Urology

A Practical Guide

Second Edition

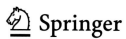 Springer

Editors
Stephen Y. Nakada
Department of Urology
University of Wisconsin
School of Medicine and Public Health
Madison, WI, USA

Sutchin R. Patel
Department of Urology
University of Wisconsin
School of Medicine and Public Health
Madison, WI, USA

ISBN 978-3-031-05539-3   ISBN 978-3-031-05540-9   (eBook)
https://doi.org/10.1007/978-3-031-05540-9

This Springer imprint is published by the registered company Springer Nature Switzerland AG
The registered company address is: Gewerbestrasse 11, 6330 Cham, Switzerland

Contents

Chapter 1
Knowing Yourself (Edition 2)

Stephen Y. Nakada

Self-awareness

Understanding yourself, and how you are viewed by others, is not simple. In the world of organized urology, there are numerous different interactions you will have, in your clinical career, academic career, and administratively. Beyond this, of course, there are all of your personal relationships, which also eventually play a role in your professional life. I believe that the sooner you begin to acquire some self-awareness about the style, habits, and overall image you emote to others, the better you will perform in all phases.

Through trial and error, you will eventually come to several fundamental conclusions about yourself. I am not an expert in this field, and thus my statements are from my experience. For instance, are you an introvert, or an extrovert? These terms are defined in Fig. 1.1. To some extent, like everything, these categories represent a continuum. However, knowing where you sit on the curve helps you with the style of your decision-making right from the beginning.

Once grounded enough in the profession, there are several excellent reference tools to help you evaluate your style as a clinician, manager, and colleague [1]. These tools require input from others, and require you to have a network of people who will fill these forms out responsibly. Typically, great feedback is scarce, but it is typically best from co-workers, and can offer you a general profile of your personality and leadership style. When involved with professional groups and societies, 360° evaluations are a common tactic. Take these exercises seriously, as the data is very valuable. I highly recommend getting a personal profile, and numerous services offer this service. Overall, while somewhat generic, you are placed into categories, which help in several ways.

S. Y. Nakada (✉)
Department of Urology, UW Medical Foundation Centennial Building, 1685 Highland Avenue, Madison, WI 53705-2281, USA
e-mail: nakada@urology.wisc.edu

© The Author(s), under exclusive license to Springer Nature Switzerland AG 2022
S. Y. Nakada and S. R. Patel (eds.), *Navigating Organized Urology*,
https://doi.org/10.1007/978-3-031-05540-9_1

Fig. 1.1 Definition

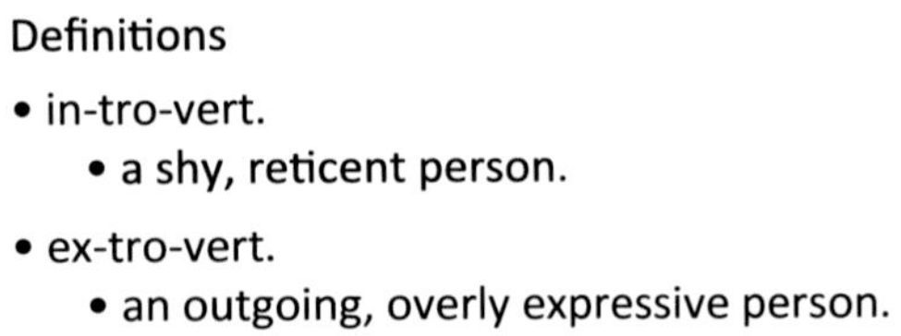

Definitions
- in-tro-vert.
  - a shy, reticent person.
- ex-tro-vert.
  - an outgoing, overly expressive person.

First, you can identify areas of improvement for yourself, and I would develop a strategy to improve your areas of weakness, and perhaps more logically avoid situations that focus on your areas of weakness. For instance, I underwent a 360° evaluation early in my career, as we performed this as a board group to help our communications in board meetings. I proved to be a poor listener, spoke too much and often appeared disinterested. Certainly the latter couldn't have been further from the truth (at least in my mind!). Regardless, focusing on listening and on faciliatory communication became a focus for me. The 360° evaluation for some was an "insult" or a "waste of time" but I saw it as a valuable opportunity. I have observed most leaders exhibit great levels of interest and a supportive demeanor, they are great listeners, and they can communicate a lot with an economy of words. For me what an eyeopener!

But admittedly it is not so simple. While didactic classes are helpful, your natural abilities play a role. Another, important alternate approach can be gleaned from the greatest modern golfer, Tiger Woods. When Woods entered the 2000 British Open which was held in St. Andrews, he was on track for his Tiger Slam (winning all four majors consecutively) [2]. The problem was that there are a record number of sand traps at St. Andrews, and Woods was a mediocre sand player by his standards. One approach would be to improve his sand play, but the key strategy was that he did not hit his ball in a bunker all week and won the tournament by a good margin. Mr. Woods avoided bunkers and opted for more difficult shots into greens, which was a strength of his game. The lesson is, even after improvement, one should select situations to exploit areas of strength and avoid situations that focus on one's weaknesses. For instance, I have learned to position myself for "delivering the message" which is a strength, rather than try and create opportunities for me to "collect the feedback." This is better assigned to someone else more naturally gifted at this whenever possible.

Priorities

Prioritization seems logical and simple, but in truth it is one of the harder things to do effectively. The challenge is how to prioritize what we set out to do, and how we use those priorities to create and *execute* a plan for our careers moving forward. The execution of prioritization relates to organized urology in this way: if you seek to be an academician focused on bench research, or a physician executive leader, or an

Fig. 1.2 The 3 P's

The 3 P's

• Performance
• Purpose
• Passion

innovator in surgical education what is the path forward, and how do I get on that path? Or maybe you just want to be the best practicing urologist you can be, or practice the least urology you can. I strongly believe all of these paths require the same fundamental starting point. Performance, purpose, and passion are my "3Ps" to success in prioritization and execution, and I have not identified anyone else coining this phrase, so for now it goes unreferenced (Fig. 1.2).

It is misguided to start out of the gate wanting to be an academic urologist, without being a great clinical urologist first. More importantly, the same goes for all paths. Want to do less urology? You better be good at it. Early in one's career, performance must be prioritized, and learning and studying to become the best clinician you can be is the first priority. In some ways, this simplifies things for you, and I found in many ways my career goals were the least conflicted as a resident. How many people as residents enjoyed all aspects of urology? I believe it will be the good ones that feel that way at some point.

Finding purpose, the second P, is an emotional decision that does come to most successful urologists. Perhaps one good way to think of "purpose" is to identify something that gives you professional satisfaction, it may be a cause, or moments (certain fulfilling cases), innovative breakthrough or practice decision that allows one to develop purpose. More recently, volunteerism, supporting DEI (Diversity, Equity, and Inclusion) are also emotional "purposes" for some. For me this was minimally invasive urology, and studying, innovating in this field gave me great direction. Decision-making, or prioritizing and executing my plan made sense, and my career became focused on acquiring skills to get become more effective. Eventually leadership and mentoring would take priority in my career. One's priorities and thus purpose can change, or more accurately evolve, but I believe this is always not necessary. The "chairman conundrum" is a great example. Most of us realize that the attributes that often position you to become chairman (success clinically and in research, a national reputation) hardly prepare you for the roles of mentorship and personnel management which are vital to this role. You can add social and emotional awareness to that list as well! Moreover, business and finance training (MBA, MHA, MMM) are degrees designed to prepare administratively, and only recently have younger faculty pursued these opportunities.

The last P, passion, is typically the most elusive. I believe passion is the ticket to extraordinary success, if you seek this. What does passion do, positively for you and your career? It lengthens the workday, it decreases your fatigue, it explains taking extreme measures to achieve success, and it explains unrelenting behaviors. This enables one to produce more than expected, or even more than is wise. George Bernard Shaw said, "when I was young, I observed that I failed 9 out of 10 times.

So, I decided to work 10 times as hard." Passion leads to followers, and followers leads to a following, which are often good things. Alternatively, this can lead to an unbalanced life, and more importantly lead to burnout and broken relationships (see Chapt. 17). As such, balance plays a role, but I would not call it a priority in this paradigm. To summarize, I believe prioritization is an evolving process and requires ongoing check-ins with your ongoing self-awareness.

Relationship Management

There are three general relationships you will have in your career: with your boss or superiors, with your colleagues, and with your subordinates (Fig. 1.3). The modern era has led us to see this traditional separation to be dwindling, but it is my belief that while in the technical sense this distinction remains, how you manage these relationships has changed dramatically. The power differential, or management of subordinates, has become critical, and for most reading this book, this aspect will expand in size and scope. Potentially this situation is a veritable minefield. Let's review these three general relationships, and some strategies to navigate them.

Bosses

Starting with your boss, here are four reasonable initial pillars to work off: (1) show up early, (2) have a list, (3) show appreciation, and (4) value growth opportunities. What does your boss do that you don't? What can you learn from that? What are his/her weaknesses?

In general, I have viewed time with my boss as opportunity, and generally a little extra time never hurts. Thus, if I have a scheduled 4:30 pm meeting, I will arrive at 4:20 pm or so, no earlier, no later. That way, if early, I get extra time or allow my boss to finish with me earlier. If the meeting does start on time, it gives me time to relax, potentially mingle with his staff, which is also beneficial. I believe faciliatory, or collaborative-type relationships are best, and nowhere does that work better than with one's superior.

Fig. 1.3 Three general relationships in your career

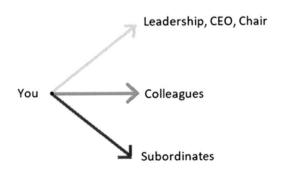

Typical List for Discussion
- Secure approval of new staff consideration[*]
- Review current funding priorities
  - Clinical education nurse
  - Research assistant
  - Data management
- Does he need me to lead this new search committee?
- Any ideas for outreach strategies

Fig. 1.4 Typical list for discussion

I always have a list of topics, that I am prepared to cut short, depending on how the meeting goes. I will prioritize these, and in fact if a topic has to be tackled I will asterisk it (Fig. 1.4). The conversation is two way, so I will often check-in first, asking if there is anything that my boss needs to talk about. If yes, I am immediately assessing my list and priorities. In discussions led by the boss, I try to use the word "we," and try and be patient, and to offer help, as well as to as clearly and simply as possible relate to the boss things that I might need to accomplish whatever the mission is.

For every good deed, there must be appreciation. I have found being appreciative is a key trait to have, and one should begin to see challenges, or assignments as opportunities rather than chores whenever possible. If you naturally cannot do this, at least recognize this and begin to reframe your outward approach. There are many opportunities for growth when "leading up," and learn to value and embrace those. Beyond the project, trust, connections, and better opportunity are around the corner. Avoid the mentality that you are somebody's "trash can." I have found that persistent growth, or daily self-improvement may alter, or in fact improve your final plan, as you may not even know what the ceiling is for your potential (see Chap. 21).

Finally, growth opportunities must be part of the plan, so knowing your own skillset will help you follow your growth opportunities. I would be clear about the growth opportunities you seek, just be consistent and concise. For example, "I am interested in leadership opportunities at the system level" is simple and clear enough. Or, "if you need someone to lead a task force on funds flow I have the bandwidth to do it" is another feasible verbiage. Regardless, a lot can be learned from the boss; I observe strengths, weaknesses, tactics, and style. Aside from adapting to the leadership model that is emoted, this relationship offers the chance to learn and observe an approach on a larger scale.

Colleagues

While theoretically the most comfortable relationship, relationships with your colleagues are always changing and can become complex. Logically it makes sense to give support, share as much as you can, and measure up. Your colleagues provide the safest haven to assess your style and make modifications. As well, study your colleagues closely; how do they relate to others? How do they use their connections? These are indeed valuable lessons. Certainly some element of competition occurs with your colleagues. This is often "trial by fire," and generally the nod goes to the skilled, collaborative colleague rather than the "loner."

Moreover, the intrigue of your relationships to colleagues is that these are truly a matrix. As you or they advance, you can rise into boss status or drop into subordinate status quickly. The old adage, be nice to the people on the way up as you will see them on the way done is very true. This can be driven by governance (becoming President for a term in an organization) or from an experience standpoint, or by chance. As a result, identify how you handle these "changes." I recommend you seek to evolve to a "congratulatory, or champagne toasting" style rather than a jealous style. There really is little benefit to the latter. I had a great urologist colleague that I had worked with for 6 years prior to me becoming urology chief. Whenever I wasn't sure what to do with a case or needed clinical advice, I would page him and ask his advice, as he was based at another hospital. Finally, in my second year as chairman, he pulled me aside and asked me to stop paging him to ask him about tough cases. When I asked why, he said, "it scares the daylights out of me every time I see your direct line on my pager!" This is a good lesson I learned about the personal dynamics of changing status with your colleagues.

Subordinates

Clearly more effective interactions with your "direct reports," subordinates, and trainees are where the money is today. Caveat emptor, there are many complexities here. I highly recommend all professionals take some formal unconscious bias training. The world is changing rapidly, and even teachers of the training course admit to subtle indiscretions regularly! Meaning well is not enough today, in today's world of extensive social media (see Chap. 16). First realize to the best of your ability how you are perceived as a leader. Are you hierarchical, a good listener, and good communicator? How are you going to know this? There are the 360° surveys, so take them whenever you can. Direct feedback helps, but I honestly believe that "constructive feedback" is often a scarce commodity. Remember, people will be nicer to you as a boss than if you were a colleague; it is a certainty, it is human nature. A good rule of thumb in managing down: seek respect, but not more than that. Or put another way, there are social limitations to your leadership of a group that should not disappoint you. Whenever we recruit or interview new job candidates, I always ask my administrative team for their feedback. This is part of the reason they are involved in the interview day, with transfers to locations, or at breakfast or lunch. The reason for this is that how candidates treat the staff is quite telling to me. It is one thing to interview with me, or the other leaders. In fact, for the candidate this is the time of "managing up," and is certainly an important skill that we have already discussed. On the other hand, interactions with staff regarding payment of travel expenses, details of the visit, answering emails, and complaints about the travel glitches are all evidence of behavior that relate to "managing down." You would want this information as well, of course. One year, we were interviewing a candidate who was terrific on paper, and the leadership and faculty were impressed. However, once I asked my administrators about this person, they related a completely different story. Unresponsive to emails, accusatory nature, and even simply rude. We decided not to hire this individual, and subsequent history would say that this was the right decision.

I have learned a lot in this area, and my advice is to seek clarity in your interactions. While challenging, this approach will help you and those around you to work better with you. Moreover, the clearer explanation of goals and plans will help you direct yourself, which is not always easy to do. As such, relationship management should evolve into a "zero hierarchy" model in the perfect world. Yet we do not live in a perfect world. I do note that in time I can place trusted subordinates in the colleague category, and vice versa. More importantly, with time you should recognize and embrace a time when your boss moves you into the colleague category. You will know when this happens, and for many of you it will, particularly if you have an enlightened leader.

Key Points

1. Do you understand what makes you truly happy professionally? Seek roles that add to your job and life satisfaction.
2. Do you know your strengths and weaknesses? Focus on positioning yourself to use your strengths, but also create a checklist of ways to improve your weaknesses, as well as ways to minimize exposure of those weaknesses.
3. Once you know yourself well enough, it makes sense to partner with people who have different skillsets than you.
4. First focus on being the best clinician you can be. Next, identify your long-term priorities and focus on opportunities that lead to success with those priorities.
5. Make a list of all the people you have a professional relationship with, and assess your rapport with these individuals. Do you prefer "leading up," working more with colleagues, or mentoring your direct reports? Measure your progress in these three fundamental areas and create a timeline of success.
6. Seek clarity of purpose and clarity in your communication style.

References

1. https://birkman.com/personality-assessments-leadership-development.
2. https://www.gsb.stanford.edu/exec-ed/programs/executive-program-leadership.
3. https://www.golf.com/tour-and-news/tigers-40-biggest-moments-no-6-completing-tiger-slam-2001-masters.

Chapter 2
Interview Skills

Sara L. Best

Abbreviation

CV   Curriculum Vitae

Congratulations! You've sent out feelers for jobs and have identified an organization with whom you share a mutual interest in exploring a potential partnership. While preparation of a curriculum vitae and email conversations can be accomplished with careful consideration and the opportunity to revise your presentation of yourself and your accomplishments, the "live interview" process is often stressful to applicants because many aspects of it are seemingly beyond your control. Fear of the unpredictable and your ability to respond to it in a way that favorably represents your abilities and personality can be anxiety provoking, but it is important to perform well in the interview process. A recent study by Kalina and colleagues reported a survey of trauma surgeons and found that "personality and likeability" were the most desired qualities in new hires [1]. And as they say, there's no second chance to make a first impression.

The good news is that while human interaction can be spontaneous, many aspects of a surgical faculty interview are actually predictable and something you can and should prepare for ahead of time. The following chapter suggests strategies for preparation.

Be Prepared

Preparing for Questions About Yourself

The same strategies used in the preparation for residency and fellowships interviews apply now. You will have updated your curriculum vitae in the application process but now is a good time to refresh yourself on its contents. Be prepared to discuss any research you have participated in, any leadership roles you have held, or

S. L. Best (✉)
Department of Urology, University of Wisconsin School of Medicine and Public Health, 1685 Highland Ave MFCB 3rd floor, Madison, WI, USA
e-mail: best@urology.wisc.edu

© The Author(s), under exclusive license to Springer Nature Switzerland AG 2022
S. Y. Nakada and S. R. Patel (eds.), *Navigating Organized Urology*,
https://doi.org/10.1007/978-3-031-05540-9_2

anything else that appears in your CV. Discussion of these topics is your time to shine! After all, you know your own experiences better than anyone so be fluent on these topics so you can demonstrate your enthusiasm, experience, and confidence. Make sure you've received your schedule of interviews ahead of time and have researched those people you will meet with so you have a general idea of their clinical and administrative roles as well as their research interests if pertinent to your job search. People are likely to search for common ground to discuss with you and you may be able to predict topics that may come up or even steer the conversation to mutual interests. For example, if you are meeting with a potential colleague with a lab that focuses on prostate cancer, and you have a publication on your CV pertaining to prostate cancer, you may be asked questions about this work. By preparing ahead of time, you have an opportunity to refresh your memory about a project you may not have thought of in some time, as well as know that your interviewer may be more knowledgeable than the average urologist about the topic.

You can also brainstorm ahead of time about potential questions you might be asked and how you would answer them. The goal of this preparation is to avoid being caught off guard, as few of us perform our best when that happens. Some general questions are to be expected over the course of any interview visit, both for the institution to "break the ice" to start a conversation and to learn more specifics about you. Some version of questions like the following are worth preparing your thoughts about before each interview:

What got you interested in our program?

What are you hoping to find in a practice?

What types of surgery/disease states are you most interested in?

Where do you see yourself in 5/10 years?

What do you like to do in your free time?

As previously mentioned, institutions are very motivated to hire the "right candidate" for the job as faculty departures/replacements are both disruptive and expensive. They want to know if you will adequately fill the role they are recruiting for as well as whether you might be dissatisfied doing so.

Questions that ask you to identify your own strengths and weakness are also common. Try to come up with a few anecdotes you can fall back on to illustrate your strengths, be they success in a leadership position, accomplishment of a research project, or even personal achievements like training for a race if they show your ability to set goals and accomplish them with hard work. Similarly, the ability to work in a team is important in physician hiring, so those experiences are also valuable to point out [2]. Citing our own weaknesses is harder so it's even more important to think this one through before being asked. The classic response of naming something often viewed as a strength like it is your weakness "e.g., I stay up too late working" is suboptimal and may not be accepted. We all have weaknesses and failures and identifying an example as well as how you have worked to overcome it is the goal. Perhaps you aren't great at answering your email because you always check it between cases while walking in the halls, but you've worked to set aside 10 min at the end of the day to review all the messages you received that day and answer them if needed. You want to appear as a person subject to the normal foibles of humankind but who is self-aware and working hard to overcome these limitations.

As you are preparing for the interview process, keep in mind that federal law prohibits prospective employers from asking questions that may facilitate discrimination in several realms. The U.S. Equal Employment Opportunity Commission prohibits unfair treatment because of race, color, religion, sex (including pregnancy, gender identity, and sexual orientation), national origin, age (40 or older), disability, or genetic information. While it may be unlikely for someone to ask you explicitly what your age or ethnicity are, in practice, the "getting to know you" aspect of the interview process may contain less explicit yet still potentially illegal questions. Institutions identify "finding someone who is a good fit" as a critical aspect of hiring and the temptation to try to categorize applicants can be strong. For example, while it is unlikely someone would ask you "Are you pregnant?", trying to "get to know someone" by asking them if they have a family may seem natural to many interviewers, though it may be illegal. And while it is strictly illegal to ask someone if they are a U.S. citizen, a similarly banned question like "Did you grow up around here?" may be well intended but provide the same kind of banned information. Think ahead of time how you would like to respond should someone ask you a potentially illegal question. While employers are banned from asking illegal hiring questions, you are welcome to share whatever information about yourself you wish to as you yourself are trying to ascertain how well you would fit in to the work environment. So you could choose to answer, or you could decline or ask "Why do you want to know?"

You also want to ensure you are scheduled to meet with everyone who is critical to the hiring decision on both sides. You will want to interview with the Chair and any subspecialty leadership pertinent to your practice plus a variety of other potential partners. Urologists with certain practice types may find it helpful to meet with non-urologist physicians, for example, the director of the children's hospital or gynecologists performing incontinence procedures.

Prepare to Ask Questions About the Job/Program

Interviewing is a two-way flow of information and this is also your opportunity to learn about a position to determine if it meets your needs. For each place you visit, you should make a list of questions you would like to have answered and determine who among the people you meet with can best answer each. Majority of interviews will see the interviewer asking you at some point if you have any questions, so have some prepared as it can make you appear disinterested if you have none.

Resist the temptation to ask about salary and call schedule early in the interview process. While these are certainly important to your job decision, the reality is asking these questions too early may be interpreted as having suspect priorities. It is better to start by asking other questions about the position and institution and ease into money and call. Traditionally those questions were reserved for a second visit but with evolutions in culture as well as more condensed search structures, it may be reasonable to pursue these carefully in your first visit. The American College of Surgeons has a great list of other questions to consider asking [3].

You should ask how the opening came up, such as faculty retirement or departure for other reasons or growth in the patient population. Ask what expertise are they hoping to add to their practice. Use these discussions to determine what kind of applicant might best fit their needs, so that you can decide whether it suits you to fill that role. For example, if the institution's bladder cancer expert just left to become Chair elsewhere, but your passion is kidney cancer, neither you nor the institution's existing kidney cancer specialist may be happy if you show up expecting to do most of the practice's robotic partial nephrectomies. While your practice will inevitably evolve over your career, knowing how much competition you will face from your colleagues to build a satisfying mix of patients for yourself can help you prepare and obtain resources to help you achieve your goals.

On the Day of the Interview

Be prompt

Whether your interview is conducted virtually or in person, tardiness universally sends a bad message and should be avoided at all costs. Your arrival time is under your control and arriving early will also allow you to feel calmer and more prepared to show your best self. Plan your travel leaving plenty of time for mishaps and for virtual meetings, block your schedule sufficiently to ensure you will be ready for the call. The necessity of timeliness applies to all interactions with your host site including replying to emails, meeting with administrative staff/recruiters, and actual interviews with your potential colleagues.

Attitude

A survey of program directors for hepatobiliary surgery fellows reported inter-personal skills to be the most important desired skill in applicants, more so even than perceived by the applicants themselves [4]. While you don't want to pretend to be someone you're not, revealing the more enthusiastic and positive aspects of your personality is a winning strategy. Resist the temptation to complain about prior work experiences or colleagues, remain engaged, limit time on your phone to periods when you are alone if possible.

Dress

The same advice you received for residency interviews applies for faculty positions. Dress conservatively, generally a suit is a safe option. Even in this digital age, it makes sense to bring a few paper copies of your CV in a briefcase or nice folder.

After the interview

It's a relief to conclude the first visit but take time to make a few notes to yourself while your memory is fresh. What were your overall impressions? Is there anything you need to follow up on or get answered? Anyone you still need to meet? Did you "click" with anyone, in particular, who might be a good resource for follow-up questions? Did you have any unique or memorable conversations that might help cement a bond going forward? And finally, is this an opportunity worth pursing further?

Regardless of whether you are interested in the job, there is no downside to being gracious to your hosts. While it may not be the right fit for you at present, burning bridges with rudeness may limit future opportunities and urology is a small world. Thank you notes or emails are still considered the norm. These notes can be tailored to your specific conversations with your hosts and are an opportunity to communicate your interest in the position. If you had a great conversation with someone about a specific topic, feel free to mention it in your note to them. Remember, studies on physician hiring suggest employers are looking for a colleague who is personable and likable. If you are confident that it is not a good fit for you, graciously let them know so they can pursue other candidates. If, on the other hand, you are interested, the notes should convey your enthusiasm and your desire to learn more. It is also an opportunity to relate what else you need to help evaluate the position, such as an opportunity to speak to other potential partners or collaborators.

The second interview

Historically institutions would conduct in-person interviews with a panel of applicants, then the search committee would meet, determine which candidates seemed like a reasonable fit, and then offer those people the opportunity to fly out for a second time, often with their significant others. At this second visit, meetings with partners you didn't meet on the first trip can often be arranged, along with anyone else you identified as being pertinent to your decision-making. You may meet with hospital executives outside the department and traditionally a realtor would give you and your partner a tour of the town, discussing lifestyle, schools, etc. There is often another dinner with your potential colleagues that may also include spouses or partners, again with the goal of determining compatibility.

While this second interview is traditional, the COVID-19 pandemic, the travel limitations associated with it, as well as the rise in the popularity and acceptance of online meeting platforms/technology have changed the process at many institutions. Many possible permutations exist and you should get a clear understanding of the institution's approach. They might do the first round of interview virtually, then invite the top candidates to visit in person, or vice versa. Or they might send an offer letter after one set of interviews, feeling comfortable with the virtual technology and their ability to "get to know you" that way. I think it's certainly reasonable to tell an institution you are very interested in, after a first round virtual interview, that you need to see a place in person to make such a big decision, especially if it's some place you're not familiar with.

Conclusions and Key Points

The interview process is critical for both sides to determine compatibility and while stressful, the questions you are likely to be asked are predictable and should be prepared for ahead of time.

- Be very familiar with your CV's contents.
- Know how you will answer common questions including those about your strengths and weakness.
- Identify questions you need to have answered to make your job decision but tread carefully initially regarding call schedules and salary.
- Remember that personality and likeability are considered critical in the hiring process.

References

1. Kalina M, Ferraro J, Cohn S. When hiring new trauma and surgical critical care fellowship graduates, what qualities are most desirable? A survey of trauma directors and trauma program administrators. Am Surg. 2018;84(2):244–7 PMID: 29580353.
2. Aycock RD, Weizberg M, Hahn B, Weiserbs KF, Ardolic B. A survey of academic emergency medicine department chairs on hiring new attending physicians. J Emerg Med. 2014;47(1):92–8. https://doi.org/10.1016/j.jemermed.2013.08.105 Epub 2013 Dec 17 PMID: 24360121.
3. The Young Fellows Association of the American College of Surgeons. The graduating surgeon: a primer for surgical trainees, p. 22. https://www.facs.org/-/media/files/member-services/yfa/yfa_graduating_surgeon_primer.ashx.
4. Baker EH, Dowden JE, Cochran AR, Iannitti DA, Kimchi ET, Staveley-O'Carroll KF, Jeyarajah DR. Qualities and characteristics of successfully matched North American HPB surgery fellowship candidates. HPB (Oxford). 2016;18(5):479–84. https://doi.org/10.1016/j.hpb.2015.12.001. Epub 2016 Feb 18. PMID: 27154813; PMCID: PMC4857058.

Chapter 3
Curriculum Vitae Preparation

Margaret A. Knoedler

Introduction

The curriculum vitae (CV) is your opportunity to provide a favorable first impression when applying for a job. From layout to content, your CV should be a clean and concise story of your professional life. It should include your education, skills, experiences, academic pursuits, and achievements, arranged in a chronologic and comprehensive manner [1]. It should be easy to read with short explanations of specific experiences. You don't need to write an entire paragraph about each volunteer experience you participated in. The goal is to be both substantive and concise [1]. To create an elegant CV, think of your task as telling a narrative. It is the history of your career so far. The cover letter and interview will be your opportunities to say where your career is going [1].

Even beyond the job search, it is important to keep your CV current [2]. The CV is oftentimes needed when trying to obtain a promotion, when giving presentations at meetings or grand rounds, and when applying for grants. It can also help you keep track of your achievements, skills, and experiences. So instead of thinking of your CV as a holiday decoration, taken out once per year and then returned to the attic, instead think of it as your coffee maker: used often, and worth frequent maintenance.

This chapter will outline a general approach to crafting a CV, specifics on what information to include and not include, and tips for making your CV stand out (in a positive way).

A CV is not a Resume!

A CV is not the same as a resume. A CV is comprehensive in its detailing of your history while a resume is a highlight of your experiences and skills in one to two

M. A. Knoedler (✉)
Department of Urology, University of Wisconsin School of Medicine and Public Health, 3rd Floor, 1685 Highland Ave, Madison, WI 53705, USA
e-mail: knoedler@urology.wisc.edu

© The Author(s), under exclusive license to Springer Nature Switzerland AG 2022
S. Y. Nakada and S. R. Patel (eds.), *Navigating Organized Urology*,
https://doi.org/10.1007/978-3-031-05540-9_3

pages. Coming out of training, your CV may be only one to two pages, but as you progress through your career, your CV may be over 20 pages [1].

Background Research

Writing a CV may sound like a daunting task. There is a paucity of literature on how to write a physician-specific, let alone a urology-specific, CV. Fortunately, you have this chapter! Furthermore, take advantage of the other resources available to you. Start by looking at examples from colleagues. Look at other urologists' CVs: what is included, what is emphasized, etc. Department Chairs, residency program directors, and residency coordinators have looked at a fair number of CVs over their many years managing faculty or resident recruitment. They are a great resource for ideas as well as reviewing your CV to provide suggestions or proofreading. Many places have created a CV institutional template for employees to use. See if you have access to one. They often have standardized formatting and organization, so you do not have to start from scratch. There are also many standard formats online to choose from.

Content

Consider the audience of your CV. Identify who will be looking at your CV and tailor the CV to the position you are seeking. Emphasize the most important information by placing it earlier in the document [3]. Below are the sections that should be included in the CV. The cover letter is separate and precedes the CV. It is only briefly mentioned here. The CV always starts with personal details followed by education, but the subsequent sections can be rearranged to emphasize your specific goals.

Cover letter

The first page is independent from the CV. The cover letter gives you the opportunity to bring your accomplishments to life [4]. It mentions the role you are applying for, provides an introduction to yourself, and why you are applying for the position [5].

Personal details

Include your full legal name and abbreviated qualifications. Don't forget the MD or DO! You worked hard for that degree. Providing your pronouns (i.e., they/them/theirs, he/him/him, and she/her/hers) is an option to avoid gender assumptions. If you choose to include them on your CV, they should be in the line under your name [6]. Address, telephone number, and email address are included next. This should be professional contact information, not personal [5].

Education

This is a list of your education and training in reverse chronologic order with the most recent accomplishments first. This includes college, medical school, residency, fellowship, as well as any other post-graduate training. Name of the institution, degree received, and dates should be included [3].

Professional or teaching appointments

Include current position held as well as any other positions held after training. Include dates as well as city and state. If currently in residency or fellowship, this section may not be included. But, if you had any gaps between undergraduate and medical school and held a non-medical position for a substantial length of time, you may want to add a section titled Work Experience to highlight these accomplishments [7].

Certification and licensure

List and give dates for each. If you are not yet board certified, state where you are at in the certification process [3]. To be board certified in Urology, one must pass the Qualifying (Part 1) Examination, colloquially referred to as the written boards, as well as the Certifying (Part 2) Examination, referred to as the oral boards [8]. One cannot claim to be "board certified" until after they have passed both examinations.

Honors and Awards

List your honors and awards along with the year granted. This can include awards received both in education as well as work [5]. List the most recent first.

Research and publications

Cite the presentations and publications that you have written or prepared. These should be in the same format as they appear in a journal, including the Pubmed ID number when available [5]. This section can be divided into sub-sections depending on its depth. For academic urologists, this section tends to be longer. Examples of sub-sections include peer-reviewed journal articles, editorial comments, book chapters, posters, local presentations, national presentations, and invited lectures.

Professional society memberships

List the societies that you belong to as well as any leadership positions held.

Personal interests

This section helps the reader remember that you are, in fact, an interesting and well-rounded individual. Rather than simply listing extracurricular activities, demonstrate why you do them and what you have gained from the experiences [5]. This section often prompts questions from interviewers so make sure the experiences represent you and you are comfortable talking about and expanding on them.

<u>Formatting</u>

The CV content should be easy to read: clean and concise. Busy formatting with multiple lines, different fonts, or overuse of **bold** or *italics* distracts the reader from the goal of the CV, which is to learn about you. Bullet points are rarely used in a CV, even though they are common in a resume [3]. Use 11 or 12 type size and 1.5 inch margins [2]. Number pages, this is especially important if your CV is long. Additionally, the CV should be converted to a PDF format before sending out electronically [4]. If you neglect this step, all the time spent on formatting may be lost when opened on a different computer platform. When printing your CV, only use white paper and preferably on a heavy cardstock. A colorful CV is not how you want people to remember you.

Succinct descriptions

When describing professional experiences or employment, using incomplete sentences is acceptable [3]. This is not the place to wax eloquently about the relationship you had with every patient you encountered during a volunteer experience. Use incomplete sentences and keep the structure of your phrases consistent throughout the document [3]. Make sure to use the same tense throughout your CV.

Example:

Vaccine Clinic Coordinator

Obtained detailed medical history from patients
Administered vaccines
Coordinated volunteers

What not to include

The CV has limitations. The high school you attended and the athletic awards you received during high school may be important to you but are not relevant on your CV. Education and accomplishments should start in college and beyond. Although common on a resume, objectives are not included in the CV [7]. The cover letter is where you can express your career goals and interest in the position.

You want to put your best foot forward. Do not include reasons for leaving previous positions or expected compensation. Except for very specific circumstances, you should not list personal health problems or disabilities [4]. Exam scores also do not need to be included in the CV. References will be included separately in your application and do not need to be mentioned on the CV.

EDIT EDIT EDIT

Once again, your CV is the first impression a prospective employer has of you. Don't be sloppy. There should not be any typos or misspellings in the CV. Have multiple people review the CV for content as well as grammar and layout. Colleagues and mentors in the field have looked at many CVs and have a sense of what makes a standout CV and what comes off as unprofessional.

Final Thoughts

Start your CV early and keep it up to date. It is a living document that will evolve throughout your career. Having a strong foundation with clean, concise structure, and wording will allow you to make an excellent first impression when applying for a job and beyond.

Helpful Hints

- Write your CV early and keep it up to date.
- Know your audience. Identify who will be looking at the CV and tailor your CV to the position.
- Quality over quantity. Concise, accurate language, and formatting.
- Proofread, proofread, proofread. Get feedback from multiple sources, no typos or misspellings.
- Convert your CV to PDF format before sending out electronically.
- Print your CV on white cardstock paper and have a copy on hand during your interview.

Key Points

- Avoid busy formatting. Keep the font the same throughout, do not overly use **bold** or *italics*.
- Don't switch tenses throughout the CV. This is distracting and detracts from the content.
- Stay simple and concise. Avoid overly wordy descriptions.
- Use abbreviations judiciously. Not everyone knows that UW stands for University of Wisconsin.

References

1. Murphy B. CV writing 101: tips for medical residents entering job market. American Medical Association. June 11, 2020. https://www.ama-assn.org/residents-students/transition-practice/cv-writing-101-tips-medical-residents-entering-job-market. Accessed 12 Oct 2021.
2. Woo R, Krawczyk Oman JA, Byrn L, et al. Writing the curriculum vitae and personal statement. J Emerg Med. 2019;57(3):411–4.
3. Creating a standout CV. American Medical Association. https://www.ama-assn.org/residents-students/career-planning-resource/creating-standout-cv. Accessed 12 Oct 2021.
4. The 5 things an employer is looking for in a resident's CV. American Medical Association. December 2018. https://www.ama-assn.org/residents-students/transition-practice/5-things-employer-looking-residents-cv. Accessed 12 Oct 2021.
5. Agha R, Whitehurst K, Jafree D, et al. How to write a medical CV. Int J Surg Oncol (NY). 2017;2(6): e32.
6. Kohler, C. Should I put my pronouns on my resume? TopResume. https://www.topresume.com/career-advice/pronouns-on-resume. Accessed 9 Nov 2021.
7. L'Heureux D. Curriculum vitae overview. Emergency Medicine Residents' Association. Accessed 18 Nov 2021.
8. Initial Certification. The American Board of Urology. https://www.abu.org/certification/initial-certification. Accessed 20 Oct 2021.

Chapter 4
Finding the Right Job

E. Jason Abel

Before you apply for a job, it is important to spend some time and honestly evaluate how you would envision your ideal future career. Every young doctor has different aspirations for his or her career. The first step should be introspective, to define, and prioritize what you value most. Because the ideal job is completely different for each individual, I found it helpful to write down a description of my ideal job as a starting point. This description evolved significantly as I gained experience and insight. However, many of my initial thoughts as a resident remain important in my current job.

Many books about philosophy, religion, and leadership are written with the sole intent of helping readers look inward to define goals. The importance of personalizing your approach to finding a job cannot be overstated since there is tremendous variability among careers. Your skills, talents, and priorities are unique. Likewise, your career path will be unique. Start as early as you can during and write down your thoughts.

"What is your ideal job?" Having your individual ideal job description helps to focus your job search and strategy. More importantly, your personal list of career goals is tremendously important and will focus you when you are negotiating and making decisions. At times, most trainees feel like they do not know enough about life as an attending urologist to make all the decisions about their future, which is a reasonable observation. However, you are the only one who is uniquely qualified to describe your ideal future career. Throughout your training, you have undoubtably seen countless examples of the positive and negative aspects of medicine and it is probably easy for most residents and fellows to list examples of certain things that they would like to include (or avoid) in their future practice.

Although it is likely that only a few important factors will truly sway your decision, it may be easier to develop a comprehensive description and then prior-

E. J. Abel (✉)
Department of Urology, University of Wisconsin School of Medicine and Public Health, Madison, WI, USA
e-mail: abel@urology.wisc.edu

© The Author(s), under exclusive license to Springer Nature Switzerland AG 2022
S. Y. Nakada and S. R. Patel (eds.), *Navigating Organized Urology*,
https://doi.org/10.1007/978-3-031-05540-9_4

itize. The list below includes some topics to consider as you develop a career plan. This list is not meant to be inclusive and you may want to include other features. Make sure to include your thoughts about how your first job will impact your ultimate career goals. After you have had time to develop your thoughts, discuss your ideas and seek input from your mentors, family, and friends. Try to prioritize which aspects of a job are most important to you and challenge yourself to clearly define your goals.

Planning Your Career in Organized Urology

LOCATION: What geographic location and practice setting will be ideal?

CLINICAL: What type of clinical practice will be rewarding for you?

RESEARCH: How important is it to include research in your future career? What resources will you want and what will success look like for you?

TEACHING: Do you want to teach residents and fellows?

FINANCIAL: How can you maximize your financial compensation? At what level of compensation will you be satisfied?

PERSONAL: What are the thoughts of your partner, family and friends?

WELLNESS: What elements of physician wellness are important to you?

LOCATION: Geographic location is an important factor for everyone to consider, especially since there is a limited amount of desirable jobs in any location at a given time. Of course, it may be easier to find a job if you are willing to look broadly, so it helps to be as open-minded as possible. Also, remember that it is not uncommon to change jobs as opportunities become available. Even if a specific geographic location is critical to you, it is wise to consider all the regional opportunities so that you can make an informed decision and understand your ability to negotiate in your future job.

In addition to geographic location, you will want to consider whether you want to be in a larger or smaller practice? In a more rural, small city, or urban environment? In a private practice setting or at an academic institution?

CLINICAL PRACTICE: A "typical" urology practice in organized medicine is almost impossible to define. When comparing two urologists that received identical training, their clinical practices in organized medicine may be completely different. What type of practice will be rewarding for you? Keep in mind that options are evolving and the practices of today will change.

As a resident or fellow, you likely observed several successful clinical practices. I remember noticing how talented my mentors were in the operating room and how well they communicated with patients. Other factors to consider include:

- How many patients will be in your catchment area and what are the needs of those patients? Are there insurance patterns or other barriers that enable or prevent your practice from growing?

- What type of team do you want to help support your patients? Physician assistants, nurse practitioners, nurses, and medical assistants play vital roles in many practices to help you provide excellent care.
- Is your employer going to market your expertise? If you are trying to build a new program, you might need to gain exposure especially in competitive markets that have established referral patterns.
- Are there adequate facilities for your future practice? For example, having urodynamics facilities, a surgical robot or a pediatric hospital may be important for your success. If these are not available, will your leadership support the development of facilities?
- What is your ideal amount of time to spend each week in the clinic and operating room?
- How important is it to you to have a flexible schedule or be able to take long vacations?
- Will you work at one hospital? Many urologists travel to different locations or see patients at outreach sites, which translates into more commuting time.
- How will on-call responsibilities impact your job?
- Do you want to focus your practice or subspecialize within urology? Although it is becoming popular in large modern urology groups, sub-specialization is not always possible or preferable especially early in your career. Your ability to focus clinically is contingent on leadership decisions and the willingness of your partners to provide complimentary services.
- Do you want to see a large proportion of patients with complex problems? Surgeries that are more complex can be rewarding but also may be unpredictable and take time from scholarly activities. Rounding on inpatients is also labor intensive especially when you have to travel to several hospitals.

Most young urologists are eager to become clinically busy. However, it is possible to become "too" busy clinically, which may affect your career development negatively. The definition of too busy is different for everyone, which is why it is helpful to define your career goals upfront but try to be honest based on an ideal environment for the description.

RESEARCH: How important is research for you? What resources will be important and what will success look like for you individually in the future? Exposure to basic science, translational, clinical, and health services research is common at urology training programs. Many graduating residents and fellows will include research in their careers. Research involvement improves understanding of clinical problems and has the potential to improve patient care, but it also requires dedication and sacrifice. In order to make scientific progress and improve treatment of urologic conditions, it is critical for Urologists to be actively involved in research. However, with changes in health care, there is always pressure for more clinical productivity, limiting time for research.

If you decide to include research in your career, you will need a strategy to find the right job. How prepared are you to do research independently? Will you need a lab for basic or translational research? Do you want to participate or design in clinical trials? Will you need research assistants to help in lab or with clinical or health services research? How will you identify an institutional mentor? Will the resources of a major research institution benefit you? Will you apply for a career development grant as a bridge to independent funding? Above all, you should prioritize how important research is to you. Many successful researchers in urology took jobs early in their career with fewer clinical responsibilities that allowed them to focus and develop their expertise.

TEACHING: Helping to train the next generation of urologists can be one of the most rewarding parts of a job in organized urology. However, teaching is not for everyone. Although most institutions are now recognizing the importance of teaching, education is time intensive and can still go unnoticed by promotion committees. How important will training others be for you in your future?

FINANCIAL: Compensation is an important consideration for any job. There are several sources of information about urologist salaries including the Association of American Medical Colleges (AAMC) and Medical Group Management Association (MGMA). Keep in mind that differences in benefits packages or total compensation is much less transparent. There are large differences in retirement benefits (some institutions offer pensions or matching funds, etc.) and insurance packages. Other institutions may provide funds for your family's college education or low-cost mortgages. Benefits packages are unique to each job but can provide significant value beyond salary support.

Student loan debt is significant for many young doctors. If you have student loans, some institutions will provide assistance in repayment. If you are involved in research, there is a Loan Repayment Program through the National Institutes of Health [1]. If you work for a government or not-for-profit organization, you may also be eligible for the Public Service Loan Forgiveness (PSLF) program [2].

PERSONAL: One of the most critical elements to consider are the opinions of your partner, friends, and family. No matter where you work, your job will have a significant impact your family. Before you look for a job, it is helpful to discuss your goals in the context of your family needs and expectations. How will a new job or new location affect your family life, including their future career and educational opportunities?

WELLNESS: Achieving an acceptable work life balance is difficult for most young surgeons but is key for longevity and career success. Looking for institutions that value your wellness is important, and you should especially look for tangible examples of defined physician wellness programs. However, each young physician may define wellness differently, and it is important to consider how your future job will support your individual needs.

Job Search Strategy

It is never too early to start exploring job options, and it is important to check back occasionally because job opportunities develop continuously. The type of jobs that you seriously consider will depend completely your individual job description and opportunities.

Most specialty societies and journals list job opportunities. Openings are posted on websites including the AUA job finder [3] and at many of the urology sub-specialty organization website. However, many good opportunities are found by networking with your mentors and peers. Ask your residency or fellowship director to send you jobs postings. Make a list of institutions that will fit with your career goals and send them your CV and cover letter. It is important to be respectful but persistent. Sometimes, a follow-up email or call from a colleague will help you to find out if an institution will be hiring in the future.

INTERVIEW: The interview process will usually involve two formal sessions but may be less or more depending on the institution. There are many books written on how to optimize your interview skills [4], which may be of benefit to review. From your ideal career description, build a list of questions for each job. When you interview, try to ask thoughtful questions to the appropriate person. For example, ask your chairperson questions about how you can accomplish your career goals and talk to a department administrator about benefits packages. Asking thoughtful questions is often seen as an indicator of preparation and quality in an applicant.

Negotiating Your First Contract

After you have received a job offer (or more than one), you are generally sent the proposed terms of the job. Check over this offer carefully to see how it reflects your discussions.

Refer back to your job description, how will the proposed job align with your career goals? Most of the time, there are some items that you can negotiate.

Two things are important to realize upfront

1. This is probably your first time negotiating a contract but it is probably not their first time. It is common to feel awkward.
2. Be courteous but do not be afraid to ask for things that are important to your career. Asking respectfully will generally not be offensive. The best opportunity to ask for more resources is before you accept your first job.

Look at each item and decide whether the resources offered provides a good opportunity that you will develop the career that you envisioned. Increases in salary may be negotiated successfully, but many academic institutions have a set range for new positions. Typically, you have a stronger position to negotiate other resources in your start-up package because your successful career development is common interest for you and your employer. Occasionally, there may be other resources that are not initially offered (for example to pay for a laboratory assistant). Similarly, if you are interested in research, you may be able to negotiate more protected time than is initially offered. It is always helpful to have a lawyer review any contracts, although institutional contracts are more likely to be standardized when compared to private practice models.

Overall Advice on Seeking a First Job

Look for the best environment that fits with your career goals. Finding a fertile positive environment to begin your career can be more difficult than it seems, and some faculty leave their first job because the environment was not what they expected. One reliable indicator of a program's environment are the current and past faculty.

In my opinion, the most important part of the environment is the leadership and overall direction of the program. Have others with similar career goals been successful at that program? Is there a record of developing young faculty within that department? Look for objective examples that you will be valued and that resources will be available for your development. Your chairperson will be tremendously important to your success; organized medicine is a team sport, and you need a strong captain.

Look for an environment with broad resources that align with your interests when possible. Having collaborators and mentors outside urology will likely be a key in the future and a formal mentorship program is often helpful.

Your future will not be someone else's past or present. Urology is an amazing field, with a vibrant history of innovation and many talented surgeons leading the charge to improve medicine for the next generation. Not surprisingly, many trainees identify with individual attending physicians as role models when they envision their future practice in urology. However, it is crucial to understand that the future will demand changes and you will have to adapt your practice just as your role models adapted their practices.

As a first year resident, I watched a talented senior surgeon perform an open radical prostatectomy with tremendous precision and skill. I felt compelled to learn as much as I could, imagining that I would use these open prostatectomy skills commonly in my future career. I asked the senior surgeon how he had learned and was shocked that he had scrubbed for only a handful of open prostatectomies during his own training. His mastery of open prostate surgery was an adaptation in response to the evolution of prostate cancer treatment during his career. Interestingly, the same surgeon adapted again to use a robotic approach for prostatectomy by the time I had finished residency.

The ability to adapt is critical for success not only in clinical medicine but also for researchers, who build on the incremental knowledge of the last generation. When you are envisioning your future career, it is wise to set goals based on becoming an expert in a disease process rather than thinking concretely. Research, education, and other academic pursuits will also undoubtably change in the future. The landscape of academic medicine is changing with an implicit goal of improving patient care. The future may bring stronger competition for funding and the urologist's role within organized medicine will undoubtable change. However, changes will also provide new opportunities for talented and adaptable urologists to become leaders in organized medicine.

Key Points

- Write down and then edit a description of your ideal career goals and your ideal first job. Although it may change with your experience, it is helpful to organize and focus your thoughts.
- Seek advice from others at many levels (early and later in their career) since you will gain valuable and different insights from each.
- Look for jobs that match your career goals. Evaluate whether the environment and leadership at each job will help you to achieve your goals.
- The future of organized medicine will provide opportunities for urologists who are able to adapt to changes.

References

1. https://www.lrp.nih.gov/.
2. https://studentaid.ed.gov/sa/repay-loans/forgiveness-cancellation/public-service.
3. https://careercenter.auanet.org.
4. Yate M. Knock 'em Dead 2017: Adams Media, A division of F+W media. 57 Littlefield Street, Avon, MA; 2016.

Chapter 5
The Role of the Educator

"No significant learning occurs without a significant relationship" ~ James Comer, MD

In 1910, Abraham Flexner, changed a primarily proprietary-driven profession into a hospital-based, patient-centered, research-oriented, and education-focused profession. With the publication of the Flexner Report, the trilogy of graduate medical education (GME) was born: patient care, research, and teaching. Each of these tenants was regarded as equally important. Patient care has always been the primary focus of the medical profession while research and teaching have become increasingly more subordinate. Of the three, teaching continues to be undervalued but can be very rewarding for medical educators.

There are as many methods of teaching as there are teachers. But the model that was used as one of the earliest forms of medical instruction, was the apprenticeship model. According to ancient Egyptian papyri,[1] it started around 440 BC. The apprenticeship model has always been a very personalized approach to teaching. Even today, apprenticeship continues to be the mainstay of medical education. The long-term relationship between the mentor and the learner allows the mentor to directly observe the pupil, which, in turn enables the mentor to grasp the true needs of the learner and correct behaviors over time.

The Halstedian approach to surgical education epitomized the apprenticeship model of teaching. This Germanic style of residency training started at the Johns Hopkins School of Medicine in 1889[2] and remains the cornerstone of all surgical training programs. The folklore of this regimented program taught trainees that

---

[1] Ancient Egyptian Medicine [1].
[2] Carter [2].

B. D. Joyner (✉)
University of Washington School of Medicine, Seattle, WA, USA
e-mail: bjoyner@uw.edu

S. Y. Nakada and S. R. Patel (eds.), *Navigating Organized Urology*,
https://doi.org/10.1007/978-3-031-05540-9_5

staying up all night on call was a chance to learn more. With the Halstedian apprenticeship model "bumping into education" then, has been one of the hallmarks of all medical training.

Over time, though, this model has become impractical and unsustainable. In today's busy, volume-driven clinical environment, trainees rotate with a different mentor every day, and in some cases, several mentors a day, with little reinforcement of good behaviors and rarely time for critical feedback or self-reflection. The GME teaching mission continues to be eroded by tensions between hospital demands and the complexities of patient care. Additionally, Halsted's principles have been chipped away by scientific advancements in educational theory, new innovative technologies, as well as external and internal pressures on the clinical learning environment.

New training techniques are based on sound concepts of how motor skills are acquired. Recently, Fitts and Posner's[3] three-stage theory of motor skill acquisition has been appreciated more with the emergence of surgical innovation and high-fidelity simulation training. In simulation centers, trainees can (1) have a set schedule to learn, (2) make errors in a non-threatening environment (3) receive feedback upon which they have time to reflect on the proper techniques, and (4) discuss next steps for graduated learning. Simulation-based medical education (SBME) continues to provide a foundation upon which structured surgical training can take place intentionally, consistently, efficiently, and safely.

More academic medical centers (AMCs) are setting aside time for faculty to train residents in their simulation centers so that residents can be taught in a safe environment before they learn on patients in the operating room. In this manner, AMCs are acknowledging the value of teaching residents in simulation centers. Furthermore, AMCs are valuing faculty time to instruct trainees by providing financial support for, as well as, credit toward promotion. There are other benefits of "sim centers," including stimulating metacognition about surgical training, producing innumerable papers on the science of surgical education and certification; and allowing more integrated learning in all surgical fields.[4]

Although simulation centers are becoming more common, especially in larger AMCs, they are not standard practice for teaching all surgical ingénues. There are many barriers to creating sim centers. The most common barrier is the cost-benefit and cost-effectiveness of simulation in medical education.[5] Training faculty and then allowing them to have time to train residents in the sim center, seem cost-prohibitive but, over time, may be cost-effective because this approach seems to have the ability to decrease patient errors and improve quality of care.

In 2021, the American College of Surgeons (ACS) introduced a pilot study in video-based assessment (VBA) which is a scalable way to assess surgical technical

---

[3] Fitts [3].

[4] Lendvay [4].

[5] Maloney [5].

skills and correlate that with patient outcomes.[6] Although intended for the life-long learning credits (formerly called Maintenance of Certification), VBA may eventually be used to supplement surgical resident education, providing learners feedback and, most importantly, allowing them to reflect upon their own skill level and ways to improve.

Other challenges to surgical training, in general, include a required, shorter resident work week, higher volume, more complex patients, and an emphasis on improving efficiency and decreasing error. All of these realities take time away from teaching the learner. The process of teaching takes time. Teachers require time to identify learners' needs and time to evaluate their deficiencies; time to develop a curriculum; time to actually teach (including providing feedback); and time to evaluate the teaching process to make improvements. Taking time away from this relationship reduces the learner's experience which remains the coin of realm of educating medical professionals.

The role of the surgical educator is simultaneous to care for the patient and to teach the learner. Balancing the two can be tedious. But, with purpose, practice, and patience, teaching can be learned—and can be fun. Without caring about the patient and the pupil at the same time, the process of teaching becomes dull and the outcomes diminished.

Medical education continues to be an unfunded mandate. And, so in order to capitalize on educating trainees, we must achieve our GME mission by maximizing time and effort. In order to achieve the combined goal of caring for the patient and teaching the trainee in a time efficient manner, various strategies have been suggested.[7] According to Irby, there is a three-step teaching process that can be adapted to any clinical learning environment: (1) identify the learner's needs, (2) teach rapidly, and (3) provide feedback. Knowing these three basic steps and practicing them when a "teaching moment" arises will improve teaching performance.

The first of Irby's steps is to *identify the learner's needs*. You can do this most efficiently with the knowledge of how learning skills is acquired. Fitts's and Posner's 3-stage process of skills acquisition is related to the four psychological stages of competence, described originally by Noel Burch but subsequently attributed to Abraham Maslow[8] (Fig. 5.1).

Figure 5.1 describes Maslow's evolution from "unconsciously incompetence" to "unconscious competence"—i.e., from not knowing what is unknown, to unconsciously knowing. When a new medical student begins to learn a task (e.g., placing a Foley catheter in a male patient), she has little knowledge of aseptic technique, the anatomy of the male urethra or which catheter size to use. This student is "unconsciously incompetent"—unaware of what is not known. After a period of education and practice (*Intellectualization* in Fitts and Posner's model), the learner becomes "consciously incompetent." At this stage, the learner becomes aware of

---

[6] ABS to Explore Video-Based Assessment in Pilot Program Launching June 2021 [6].

[7] Irby [7].

[8] Four stages of competence [8].

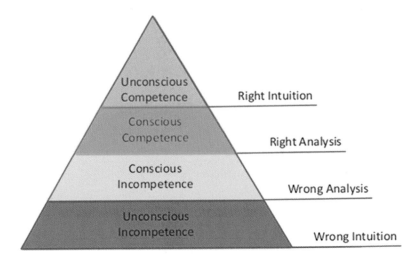

Fig. 5.1 Maslow's hierarchy of competence

what they can and, perhaps more importantly, of what she cannot do. The third stage in Maslow's psychological evolution of learning is "consciously competent." This occurs when the learner becomes aware of what to do but the steps and process are not automated; errors can occur if concentration is not maintained during the task (*Integration* in Fitts and Posner's model). With direct observation by a supervisor, at some point during this stage, the learner becomes safe to practice independently. The final stage "unconsciously competent" is gained typically after years of practice and thoughtful reflection (*Automation* in Fitts and Posner's model).

As Vaporciyan[9] points out, there is a conundrum with training any learner, but especially surgical residents: Many of those training, perform surgery at the "unconsciously competent level" whereas those being trained are dichotomous at the "unconsciously incompetent" level. That is, the master surgeon oftentimes forgets how she learned the details of a procedure and therefore, finds it hard to teach the learner who is completely unaware of the procedure, much less, the details of how to acquire the skills. As such, the first step in becoming a *master teacher* is to reduce the gap between what the *master surgeon* knows and what the *novice* does not know.

Predictably, all residents have limited knowledge and gaps (i.e., "incompetence") in their learning. When these gaps are identified, you should assess the

---

[9] Vaporciyan [9].

learner further and then focus on a "teaching moment." Irby[10] provides several teaching models that can be used to assess, and at the same time, provide an opportunity for the teaching moment to occur.

The *One-Minute Preceptor*[11, 12] is perhaps the most widely known and researched teaching method in medical education. It involves a five-step process where you should invite the learner into a conversation. During the conversation, you (1) obtain a commitment from the learner, (2) probe for underlying reasoning, (3) explain general principles, (4) provide positive feedback, and (5) correct errors and make suggestions for improvement. These five steps may seem cumbersome, and in many ways artificial because the order of the steps is not as important as the time spent understanding the learner's needs and teaching to those needs.

Activated demonstration[13] is another model that is most meaningful during a patient encounter when learners are unfamiliar with a particular problem. This model is perfect to use in the clinical setting or in the operating room. Activated demonstration occurs when the learner is given a specific assignment during which time observation of the task or procedure should occur. For example, during a hypospadias procedure, the teacher might say, "Watch the position of my wrist and the angle of the 15-blade while I perform the dissection of the glans penis to create the glans wings." Following the dissection, you *activate* the learner by asking her to describe what she observed. A brief conversation ensues, as necessary and, following the procedure, you can assign independent study and practice.

The time-honored *case presentation* is a staple in medical education, often used in the ambulatory setting or at the patient's bedside. You should be aware of the several techniques required to use this model efficiently and effectively. Essential techniques include (1) informing the patient of the transaction, (2) instructing the learner of their role, (3) physically triangulating the patient and learner with the teacher such that the patient is in the center, and (4) using the opportunity to concurrently teach the learner and inform the patient.[14, 15]

Teaching while operating, in the clinic and during patient rounds, has become more challenging due to the competing priorities in the clinical environment, which have changed dramatically over the last 100 years. Having several teaching models to fill gaps in learning allows the teacher flexibility to adapt instruction to the unique needs of each learner in an oftentimes-imperfect clinical environment which is filled with uncertainty.[16]

---

[10] Irby [10].

[11] Aaraard [11].

[12] Teherani [12].

[13] Wilkerson [13].

[14] Smith [14].

[15] Usatine [15].

[16] Irby [16].

Feedback

"Feedback" is a relatively new term, coined by flight engineers but has been adapted as a well-known educational tool used in apprenticeship models for centuries. Feedback is a personal, one-on-one verbal communication which should be used to promote good behaviors and, more importantly, to correct learner errors. Feedback is used to help the learner get to their target, which is to develop into an independent practitioner of medicine. Sometimes, though, learners take feedback as if they *are* the target! This response, of course, consciously, or unconsciously discourages the teacher from providing any feedback at all in order to avoid an uncomfortable learning environment. We shouldn't leave learners to their own devices, though, particularly the medical students and junior residents. We need to observe all learners directly and as often as possible because observation is essential to providing proper and timely feedback.

Providing *feedback* is one of the most important parts of the teaching process.[17] In the face of this statistic, the most egregious complaint learners have is that feedback is not only insufficient but inadequate. *Effective* feedback allows learners to gain the knowledge and skills they need, especially in the current shift toward competency-based education (CBE).[18] When done well, feedback achieves two seemingly opposing goals: (1) *positive feedback* for the learner whose skills or behaviors are correct and (2) *critical feedback* for the learner with misconceptions, missteps, or mistakes. These goals are unified. Together, they attempt to improve the learner's behavior for safe, independent practice.

The medical field is not alone in its inability to provide effective feedback, but it does have some unique features that may create idiosyncratic concerns in medical education. First, surgical culture is very hierarchical and, traditionally, has only provided what was once referred to as *negative* feedback. Times have changed. Negative feedback has been rebranded and is now called "critical" feedback. Critical feedback involves the act of correcting the learner's knowledge, behavior, or attitudes by using different methodologies.[19] Oftentimes, and related to the issue of our hierarchical culture, the teacher focuses not on the learners' observed behaviors but on the learners themselves. This can lead to mistrust and very bad outcomes. Therefore, be sure that your feedback focuses on the learner's *behavior* and not the learner.

Second, the Socratic Method has fallen out of favor. Before 2001, the Socratic method was a very popular way to teach during medical and surgical rounds. The Socratic method was the way in which teachers assessed the learner's knowledge and determined lapses in that knowledge. Unfortunately, in medicine, the Socratic method became known as "pimping"—a means of intimidation instead of a method of instruction. Pimping was viewed by today's learners as a way to embarrass them instead of educating them. And, even worse, it created a divide in the student–

---

[17] Veloski [17].

[18] Holmboe [18].

[19] Ende [19].

teacher relationship. Over time, trust in that relationship, so central to the apprenticeship model of teaching, was lost. That is not to say that the Socratic method should not be used. It simply needs to be approached in a different manner: by communicating the purpose—and oftentimes, using a different tone.

Third, there are lingering, misguided concepts that make both learner and teacher mistrust the feedback process. Most learners resist critical feedback because of tone but also because they have (1) misconceptions that all feedback is negative and (2) challenges with self-assessment, related to self-image. On the other hand, teachers find critical feedback exceptionally challenging because they (1) are unfamiliar with techniques of giving effective feedback and (2) are fearful of ruining the learner–teacher relationship. Algirairgri's insightful article provides us with ten tips for effective feedback and reminds us to empower learners with skills to properly receive and process feedback, regardless of whom, how, or when feedback is delivered.[20]

The final concern with providing feedback in today's medical climate has to do with the itinerate resident rotations. Before the middle part of the twentieth century, apprenticeships lasted 9 months to several years. Now, average rotations are 3 weeks, 4 at most. These brief rotations tend to create fragmented student–teacher relationships—and, consequently, fragmented learning. The key to feedback that has been shown to change behaviors is to establish a strong, trusting learner–teacher relationship. This is nearly impossible when residents are itinerant. In such settings, feedback should be provided—and is preferred by the Millennial learner, in frequent, in-person "*tweets*". During these brief conversations, you should capture a "teaching moment," using the One-Minute Preceptor or the Activated Demonstration models. Either of these—and many other teaching models, can be structured as nuanced conversations to identify gaps in the learner's knowledge, present principles, and provide feedback, as necessary. Brief unstructured conversations, like this, can direct the learner to exercise individual agency while conveying respect for them.

The foundation of effective feedback is *honesty*. Feedback should go beyond praise, which is important because it confirms for the learner what is going well. Providing positive feedback is easy to give by teachers and easily accepted by learners. The most stressful part of teaching is providing *critical* feedback. Critical feedback is essential for correcting misconceptions, missteps, or mistakes. Developing confidence around delivering critical feedback involves valuing the learner–teacher relationship, acquiring useful feedback techniques, practicing feedback as often as possible and developing confidence in feedback. Encouraging learners to ask for feedback should be part of your feedback repertoire.

---

[20] Algiraigri [20].

SMART feedback[21]

- Specific—deal with the problem at hand; don't overwhelm the learner with multiple issues.
- Measurable—the learner's level should be considered and feedback should be provided as such.
- Achievable—observe the learner and allow them to be successful by *complimenting and correcting* behaviors for their specific level.
- Relevant—feedback should relate to what they need to know for their level.
- Timely—as much as possible, and as discretely as possible, provide prompt feedback in a private setting.

Success in education can only be achieved when we are skeptical because having a critical eye forces us to look closer at the evidence—the ideal source of what we should be doing and what we could be doing better.

Hopefully, this chapter has provided you with some insight into teaching so that you might reflect on your own teaching style and commit to making durable improvements.

Twelve Tips for Medical Educators

(1) Teachers are not born. They evolve through intentional practice, and most importantly, a deliberate *desire* to teach. Good teachers emanate from and are sustained by individual commitments, like creating teaching moments, connecting with individual learners, following up with them, and watching them develop into independent surgeons.

(2) Teachers should be curious about their learners. Spend time with your learners. Get to know them better so that you might determine what they need to succeed. Feedback should start with the teacher being curious: *ask* the learner about their behavior or action. After they have responded, tell them what they did right and how they could improve. Assign reading materials, as necessary and follow-up. We all have something to teach—and, if we look beyond ourselves, we all have something to learn.

(3) Teachers are mentors. They are responsible for creating strong relationships with their learners. They should not, however, have a goal of being friends with their learners. *Friendship* and *friendly* are not the same thing. One is a noun and the other is an adjective. But the real point is that teachers should be friendly with their learners but not begin friendships with them. First, friendship eventually erodes at the learner–teacher relationship. Second, teachers cannot discipline learners when they are friend with them.

(4) Teachers should resist social media relationships with their learners. Twitter and Instagram may be the current social trends, but they are painfully blunt social constructs for doing what should be the delicate work of forming human relationships. Social media is an excellent utility for sending and

---

[21] SMART Criteria [21].

receiving data, but we are not data and relationships should not be reduced to exchange of data or binary decisions of friending and unfriending.

(5) Teachers should not ignore the broad contexts and variability of their learners. Teachers should understand their learner's preferred learning styles. For example, the Millennial learner grew up with social media. She prefers frequent, brief bursts of communication that is explicit and outcomes-oriented pointed.

(6) Teachers should attempt to appreciate their learner's diverse backgrounds and understand bias, micro- and macroaggressions, as much as possible. Unintentional, discriminatory *faux pas* can be extremely impactful and destroy trust in a relationship.

(7) Teachers should always be medical professionals in everything they do, from demeanor to dress. Our actions model essential messages of commitment to our patients—and to our learners. We do not wear our *curriculum vitae* on our forehead for patients to see. So, we should always promote messages of improving patient care, professionalism, integrity, and accountability.

(8) Teachers need to be continuous learners themselves. In this way, we can provide proper communication, feedback, and evaluations for each new generation! Take advantage of faculty development courses and workshops. Network with other specialties and read outside the medical field. These habits will allow you to expand your knowledge, especially if you apply what you learn to your specialty. There is a tremendous amount to know—and to teach.

(9) Teachers don't need to know every teaching model or academic theory. They should identify teaching models with which they feel most comfortable and learn to assiduously adapt them to the learner's needs.

(10) Teachers should always look for opportunities for professional development, especially for junior faculty who should constantly be involved with developing themselves, *first*. Progress in life-long learning and achieving promotion should be beneficial outcomes of those efforts.

(11) Teachers can make a lasting impression on their trainees. Be consistent and fair with all learners, embracing their knowledge, as well as their faults. Champion the learning process.

(12) Teachers should remember that the coin of the realm of education is experience—real, hard, honest experiences that provide trainees with knowledge and skills. We must provide them with observable and supervised experiences but residents must take time to reflect on these experiential opportunities and internalize their meaning in order to develop true wisdom.

References

1. Ancient Egyptian Medicine. Wikipedia. https://en.wikipedia.org/wiki/History_of_medicine. Accessed Oct 2018.
2. Carter BN. The fruition of Halsted's concept of surgical training. Surgery. 1952;32:518–27.
3. Fitts PM, Posner MI. Human performance. Belmont, CA: Brooks/Cole; 1967.
4. Lendvay TS, Casale P, Sweet R, Peters C. VR robotic surgery: randomized blinded study of the dV-Trainer robotic simulator. Europe PMC. 2008;132:242–4.
5. Maloney S, Haines T. Issues of cost-benefit and cost-effectiveness for simulation in health professions education. Adv Simul. 2016;1:13.
6. ABS to Explore Video-Based Assessment in Pilot Program Launching June 2021. https://www.absurgery.org/default.jsp?news_vba04.21. Accessed May 2021.
7. Irby DM, Wilkerson L. Teaching when time is limited. BMJ. 2008;336:384–7.
8. Four Stages of Competence. Wikipedia. https://en.wikipedia.org/wiki/SMART_criteria. Accessed Sept 2018.
9. Vaporciyan AA. Teaching and learning surgical skill. Ann Thorac Surg. 2016;101:12–4.
10. Irby D, Aagaard E, Teherani A. Teaching points identified by preceptors observing the one-minute preceptor and traditional preceptor encounters. Acad Med. 2004;79:50–5.
11. Aaraard E, Teherani A, Irby D. Effectiveness of the one-minute preceptor model for diagnosing the patient and the learner: proof of concept. Acad Med. 2004;79:42–9.
12. Teherani A, O'Sullivan P, Aagaard E, Morrison E, Irby D. Student perceptions of the one minute preceptor and traditional preceptor models. Med Edu. 2007;29:323–7.
13. Wilkerson L, Sarkin RT. Arrows in the quiver: evaluation of a workshop on ambulatory teaching. Acad Med. 1998;72(suppl 10):S67–9.
14. Smith AG, Bromber MD, Singelton JR, Foreshew DA. The use of "clinic room" presentation as an educational tool in the ambulatory care setting. Neurology. 1999;52:317–20.
15. Usatine RP, Nguyen K, Randall J, Irby DM. Four exemplary preceptors' strategies for efficient teaching in managed care settings. Acad Med. 1997;72:766–9.
16. Irby D, Wilkerson L. p. 385.
17. Veloski J, Boex JR, Grasberger MJ, Evans A, Wolfson DB. Systematic review of the literature on assessment, feedback and physicians' clinical performance: BEME Guide No. 7. Med Teach 2–6; 28:117–28.
18. Holmboe ES, Yamazaki K, Edgar L, et al. Reflections on the first 2 years of milestone implementation. J Grad Med Educ. 2015;7:506–11.
19. Ende J. Feedback in clinical medical education. JAMA. 1983;250:777–81.
20. Algiraigri AH. Ten tips for receiving feedback effectively in clinical practice. Med Educ Online. 2014;19:25141.
21. SMART Criteria. Wikipedia. https://en.wikipedia.org/wiki/SMART_criteria. Accessed Sept 2018.

Chapter 6
The Urologist as an Effective Administrative Leader

Edwin A. Melendez and James M. McKiernan

Urologists are uniquely equipped with the skills and experiences to serve as effective administrative leaders in the current healthcare climate. With complex healthcare challenges such as treating patients across the care continuum to identifying new, cost-effective ways to move treatment from the inpatient to ambulatory setting, the clinical subspecialty lends itself to addressing some of these broader issues in the day-to-day management of patients with urologic conditions. For example, unlike cardiothoracic surgeons who have the ability to refer to their medical cardiology counterparts, urologists are often managing patients across the surgical and medical continuum. In addition, as technological advances have emerged in the urologic field, an increasing number of cases are moving from the inpatient, operating room to outpatient, procedural spaces. As such, the practicing urologist inherently cares for patients beyond their primary urologic condition and is often incorporating innovative treatment modules that move care outside of the hospital setting. In essence, urologists are primed for some of the greatest healthcare administrative challenges by their clinical experiences alone. Clinical experience, however, is merely one facet of becoming an effective healthcare administrator.

Before advising on how an urologist can be an effective administrator it is important to review what administration entails. Traditional healthcare administration is viewed as business administration, overseeing financial or operational functions of a healthcare organization. However, this is a very narrow definition of the array of administrative roles that exist today. Both the academic urologist as well as the urologist in independent practice have a vast number of administrative roles available to them at the departmental and organizational level. Such opportunities can range from intradepartmental positions of quality assurance officer, clinical practice director, business and finance director, residency program coor-

E. A. Melendez · J. M. McKiernan (✉)
Department of Urology, Columbia University Vagelos College of Physicians and Surgeons, New York, NY, USA
e-mail: jmm23@cumc.columbia.edu

© The Author(s), under exclusive license to Springer Nature Switzerland AG 2022
S. Y. Nakada and S. R. Patel (eds.), *Navigating Organized Urology*,
https://doi.org/10.1007/978-3-031-05540-9_6

dinator, or division chief. They may also involve opportunities for larger scale administrative leadership such as department chair, hospital president, academic or clinical dean positions, chief medical officer, cancer center director, or even national or international society leadership roles in the American Urologic Association, American Board of Urology, or specialty societies. With all of these opportunities available for the aspiring urologist a brief outline of the essential skills and values required for effective administrative leadership is appropriate.

However, as a urologist in an administrative role it may not be enough to simply embrace the essential skills needed to be an effective leader. External factors such as public health emergencies and a global pandemic, including the recently experienced COVID-19 pandemic, provide heightened challenges beyond the status quo of hospital administration. In times like these, there is ambiguity, complexity, uncertainty, and volatility that require facile navigation of both hard and soft leadership skills necessary for an administrator to maintain operations and keep patients safe and well cared for. In this chapter, we will start by discussing the fundamental characteristics that differentiate an effective administrator, listing concrete strategies to being successful in an administrative role, and expanding on these strategies by highlighting takeaways specific to leading during times of crisis. We caution that the following summary is by no means complete and should serve as a starting point for further study and review.

Looking Inward

While the roles vary in scope and function, there are fundamental characteristics that differentiate an effective administrator that begin by looking inward. The most successful administrators identify their motivation for administrative pursuits and maintain a clear understanding of their own principles of leadership.

To be an effective administrative leader, you must be clear about your motivation and goals for pursuing an administrative career. As a medical professional, taking on administrative responsibilities invariably takes away from time available to care for patients or pursue academic or research interests. You must come to terms and be comfortable with the tradeoffs associated with pursuing a career in administration early on. You must have a concrete understanding about why you are pursuing an administrative role. For example, for some, taking on administrative responsibilities allows for them to effectively care and change the care for many patients rather than at the individual patient level through helping solve complex operational and strategic issues. For others, taking on administrative roles serves as an outlet to relieve stress from the day-to-day clinical responsibilities of taking care of patients. There are also instances where individuals take on administrative roles as opportunities to explore diverse interests outside of traditional academic medicine, including leadership, organizational behavior, strategy, or data analytics to name a few. This motivation may be driven by the fact that many clinicians after long periods of learning during training, feel unsatisfied with practicing for 25–

30 years with little opportunity for learning new skills. Ultimately, to be effective, you need to understand why you are pursuing an administrative career and be able to clearly articulate this.

In addition to understanding your motivation, it is important early on in your administrative career to determine your principles of leadership. These are your own core values of communication, motivation, organization, and inspiration. Such things as transparency, inspiring great performance through examples, rewarding outstanding behavior, and negative feedback in response to sub-par performance are all examples of transmitting how you will lead. Your principles may mirror your personality and your core values however, it is important for you to communicate them to members of your administrative team early on and for you to adhere to these principles in times of great stress. That is, to be consistent in your leadership values across circumstances, regardless of the "style" you must employ to address a certain issue. It is human nature to act less predictably in times of stress and stray from principles and this can lead to a team that loses trust. If your team members fail to trust their leader, they will most likely not follow that leader and a leader who looks over his/her shoulder to see no followers is no longer a leader.

Concrete Strategies

Once you have understood your reasons for pursuing administration and have a clear understanding of your leadership principles, you can begin practicing some externally-facing strategies to be more successful in the administrative role you ultimately choose. There are many "hard" skills that make a physician more effective at administration. For example, the Physician Executive Management Center survey identified a number of these skills, including: effective communication across mediums, ability to persuade, motivate and influence people, ability to lead strategic planning, computer skills and skills in finance and people management [1]. Some of these skills can be acquired through training, education, or mentorship, and without necessarily pursuing a degree in business administration. However, the softer people management skills of yourself and others are usually developed and refined through exposing yourself to relevant experiences. Below we outline some concrete strategies you can employ yourself to become a more effective administrator.

(1) Choose the right role in the right organization for you at a given time

Working for the right person is a critical success factor to being successful in any role, but particularly in an administrative role that is unstructured and requires a high degree of intrinsic motivation to tackle on a day-to-day basis. The culture of an organization or team will either create a soil for you to grow or conversely for your career to be stunted—it is important as you evaluate opportunities to gauge whether you feel that an organization and the leader you will fall under will extract your potential based on your interactions or not. It is especially paramount that young trainees become aware of the attributes they should look for in the administrative leaders of the organization that they are considering for their first job. This may include departmental, medical school, hospital, health system or group practice administration. Each will play a vital role in the early success of their career. A talented young urologist without an effective administrator and leader will be like a sailboat on the ocean without a rudder. You will be buffeted by the rough seas of academic or private practice and end up shipwrecked on a random desert island. In order to avoid this fate, in addition to identifying leadership and organizations that will extract your potential, you must also seek out an administration with leaders who are humble. Humility is generally bred from high self-esteem. Nothing is more destructive to your growing career than an environment in which the administration is formed by leaders who are abusive and resort to demeaning behavior to generate results. Abusive and demeaning behavior almost always stems from a lack of self-esteem and these leaders should be avoided at all costs.

Equally important to selecting the right boss and organization is that you select leadership roles with responsibilities that are commensurate with authority [2]. Without this balance, often you end up with a fancy title and a long list of responsibilities, but do not feel empowered or capable of achieving your goals or delivering on expectations. Upon joining the right organization or team, you must understand their vision, strategy, and goals. Remember to often re-ask what has changed so that you can continue to move towards where the organization needs to go and evolve with it or know when to move on when your values are no longer aligned with the organization.

(2) **Be willing to be uncomfortably vulnerable**

As a physician who has been trained to identify the correct multiple choice answer across the countless exams in your training or determine the correct diagnosis or treatment plan for dire patient care situations, it is a difficult prospect to be in an administrative role where there is rarely a sole, "right answer" in any of your day-to-day decisions, but rather, several viable options. As an administrative leader, while there may be situations you are comfortable addressing based on your experiences, there will be many more that you may never have encountered before and are still expected to address with confidence. It is tempting to avoid such roles and situations or consistently defer to others so that you can be more likely to be "correct" and avoid the risk of failure. It is very important to both strive for continuous learning and improvement in administrative roles and expose yourself to unknown or uncertain situations. As a medical professional entering administration, exposing yourself to areas of uncertainty may include things like volunteering to be on department committees, speaking up at meetings with your perspective and input, particularly when you disagree, or saying yes to opportunities to help solve issues where you do not feel 100% equipped to do so. It is both ok to take these opportunities on and express your vulnerability as this will allow you to gain more experience and confidence, and ultimately ensure that you are supported in these times of learning with the right mentorship from your leaders.

(3) **Be open and accessible**

Both front-line staff and administrators need a clinical resource as both a sounding board and advisor to help think through complex issues. By being an open and accessible resource for these conversations, you are developing relationships with individuals and teams who can help you solve issues you are grappling with and identify other issues to focus on. As discussed above, you are rarely going to have the silver bullet or "right answer" to every issue that you come across, and therefore it is important to build sincere relationships with various role groups early on that you can tap into to be more effective in how you approach various problems. Identifying the high-impact problems to prioritize is equally important so that you can spend your time wisely and again, improve your effectiveness as an administrator. Ultimately, front-line administrative and clinical staff often have the most valuable insights and experiences making them capable of informing administrative leaders on the most pressing issues and provide practical ideas to help solve them. In your pursuit to glean this valuable insight, you need to be present and available to staff—you need to make it very clear that you want to hear from team members without judgement and that you have time to do so. An example of this is to create a weekly "drop-in" session where you will be in your office no matter what else is going on to be available to your team. You must make it evident that you care to listen and that you are willing to learn with an open mind in these situations, regardless of your potential biases, in order to solicit honest, insightful input. Once you become an administrative leader who is known to be open and accessible, likely you will not only be more effective in your role, but people will begin to identify you for other roles as well.

(4) **Be obsessed with measuring progress**

A key feature of any effective administrator much like any medical researcher is the capacity to measure what they are trying to do. Data is a critical currency in the world of healthcare administration and when you are tasked to solve any problem or issue, it is important to figure out a way to measure the current state and set concrete targets for a future, improved state that allow you and others to objectively measure your performance. This may include measuring RVU productivity, measuring wait times on telephone lines, measuring the number of infectious complications, measuring the number of publications of a department. No effective administrator can do their job without defining the goal and measuring progress toward that goal. James Harrington captures the importance of data when he said: "Measurement is the first step that leads to control and eventually to improvement. If you can't measure something, you can't understand it. If you can't understand it, you can't control it. If you can't control it, you can't improve it." [3]. Often in healthcare, particularly in the hospital setting, it can be challenging to source the exact data you would like or more difficult than expected to have the ability to design and run your own reports independently. This can be incredibly frustrating and discouraging, but it is helpful in these junctures to know who you can go to help obtain this data. It is also critical to develop the right relationships with colleagues who can obtain data and focus on processes that matter to the organization so that your requests are prioritized. It is also helpful to use proxies for measures rather than aiming for perfection in data collection, and identifying future processes that you can design to help optimize data collection moving forward.

(5) **Identify and retain the right talent**

Perhaps the most important task assigned to physicians placed in administrative leadership roles is that of choosing and retaining strong talent. Human capital or personnel decisions are critical to the success of any organization and bad decisions made in this regard can become rapidly insurmountable. The talent in your fellow team members may be represented in clinical faculty, administrative personnel, finance team members, nurses, residents, researchers or administrative support staff. All team members play a role and no decision in this area should be taken lightly. The simplest formula for success that we have seen comes from Jack and Suzy Welch in their book entitled, "Winning." [4]. In this book they noted that team members can be categorized into 4 subtypes based on the traits of behavior and productivity with behavior being on the Y axis and productivity on the X axis. For the purposes of this discussion assume the team member is a urologist joining the practice. In category 1 we have the highly functional team player who gets along well with everyone, follows the mission of the organization and is supportive of the direction the team is going in. However, this particular doctor is having hard time building a practice and is underproductive on revenue generation and RVUs as well as academic productivity. This particular type of doctor needs administration's help and his worth the investment of time and energy. In category 2 we have the highly functional, well behaving urologist who is liked by all, supports the mission of the team and is highly productive clinically and academically. This person should be left alone by the administration to serve as an example and a mentor to others for them to aspire toward. In category 4 we find the underproductive, bad-behaving team member who undermines authority, creates unrest, wastes resources and fights the mission of the organization, while not producing results. These may be the simplest team members to identify and are often terminated prior to you becoming an administrator; however, if they have not been, an example needs to be made of them very quickly. This group is often referred to as "disruptive and underproductive jerks." In group 3 we find the most common and most important challenge in administrative leadership—the highly productive, bad-behaving team member. In every industry these individuals can be identified and they are often tolerated or even elevated into positions of great power. They will serve as a very destructive force in your organization and can act as a negative example of what will be tolerated simply because of clinical or academic productivity. It is our belief that these team members must also be removed from the organization as soon as possible in order to prevent others emulating their behavior. It may be difficult to do so in the short-term as the loss of their productivity will hurt the organization. In the long-term however, the culture of the organization and team will be far better off without them. Moreover, the role of an administrator running a team full of category 1 and 2 individuals can be a joyfully rewarding experience.

(6) **Get people in your corner**

As discussed earlier, developing important relationships early across the clinical and administrative teams is an important aspect of identifying the right problems to solve and helps you to consider novel approaches to solving them that may help you be more effective in your role. Getting people in your corner is one step further than developing strong relationships—this is getting to a place with individuals who will both advocate for and protect you. Creating such business partners and allies also provides you with informal mentorship and people to help teach you about the political climate or issues to look out for. Early in your administrative roles, you will need to identify such allies and a few things to consider in doing so include asking yourself whether you "click" with this potential ally, whether this person has some degree of insight into an area you need to learn, and whether this person has the credibility and respect in the organization to serve as a strong support to you. Such allies not only live in higher leadership roles, but are also your peers and direct reports at various levels of the organization.

(7) **Embrace your clinical roots**

Since we are discussing a medical professional such as a urologist in an administrative role, we would be remiss in not acknowledging the balance of maintaining an identity as a clinical professional and an administrator. Most successful clinical administrators are those who keep a foot in the clinical world as this gives them credibility with staff, helps them maintain a pulse on what is actually going on, and allows them to make better decisions as an administrator. Additionally, by continuing to spend time clinically, you have an easier time keeping an emotional tie to the real purpose of the organization or team and will be more likely to feel empathy for your clinical staff.

(8) **Know when to lead versus manage**

Traditionally leaders and managers are quite distinct. A leader's role is to create the long-term vision of the organization, whereas the manager is dedicated to keeping the organization following this vision. It is important to know in your administrative role when you need to operate with your management versus leadership hat. The simplest analogy that we have found to distinguish the roles of a worker, manager and leader is that of a team navigating its way through the jungle. One group is up on a ladder seeing over the tree-tops and making sure the team is navigating in the correct direction and not about to fall off a cliff. These are the leaders. Another group is literally hacking through the underbrush and blazing a trail through the jungle floor; these are the workers. The third group is sharpening the machetes and providing food and water to the workers; these are the managers. If this scenario seems too abstract then perhaps the famous quote by Peter Drucker will sum things up better: "Management is doing things right—improving operational performance, maximizing revenues, and reducing expenses while increasing artistic production values and audience appreciation. Leadership is doing the right things—setting organizational priorities and allocating human and fiscal resources to fulfill the organization's vision." [5].

Leading Through Crisis

At some point in every administrator's career, they'll be faced with a crisis. Whether this crisis is large-scale and public facing, something that is contained and private, or—as is the case with the COVID-19 pandemic—something that is experienced globally, a crisis is a time of intense stress and complexity with no one perfect solution or easy path to recovery [6]. Carlos A. Pellegrini, past-president of the American College of Surgeons, summarized this best in stating "This is not leadership as usual—this is leadership on the edge." [7]. While on edge, administrative leaders are tasked with managing the crisis, learning new lessons along the way and developing creative problem-solving strategies to keep their enterprise operational. Below we highlight some key characteristics and practices that effective administrative leaders should embody during times of crisis. Surgical administrators such as urologists have often honed these strategies over many years by facing rapidly changing and high stakes scenarios in the operating room.

(1) **Be present and lead by example**

As a clinical administrator you will be in the enviable position of the player coach. You will be asked to lead, but be given the opportunity to participate in the game as a clinician as well. This is more than half the battle because it allows you to lead by example physically through your actions rather than simply your strategy. In March of 2020, the first case of COVID-19 was confirmed in New York State and the National Guard was called in to attempt to quarantine the outbreak our health system faced during this crisis. Within 4 weeks our health system was caring for over 2,600 hospitalized patients with 762 requiring ventilator assistance. With our operating rooms closed and a dire need for redeployment, several models of real-locating house officers were proposed. Our surgical administrative leaders adopted a model of deployment involving senior surgical faculty paired with junior surgical residents entering together into the unknown crisis of COVID-19. This opportunity to lead by example infused a new found confidence into our team members that was greatly needed at a time of enormous uncertainty [8]. Clinicians in administrative leadership roles should embrace these opportunities to be present in the crisis and you will be amazed by the intangible effects it will have on those you are leading.

(2) **Communicate often and thoughtfully**

It is often said it is impossible to over communicate in times of leadership crisis. Often healthcare leaders may find themselves updating 3 or 4 different audiences in the same week regarding the same facts and feel frustrated that they are not making progress. It cannot be stressed enough how reassuring information can be even if the information is not good news. Uncertainty produces anxiety throughout the workforce, and a leader's silence will often be interpreted as bad "local" news [9]. Therefore, it's essential for leaders to consistently define reality and reinforce a clear perspective on what is happening while translating the impact for your audience. In addition to consistent communication, thoughtful and thorough communication needs to be exercised. While it may feel natural to communicate mostly action items and directives, times of crisis call for a balance between these "cold instructions" and conceptual insight in order to connect with your personnel. Providing this insight allows for your audience to buy in to the mission at hand, leading to higher efficacy in executing the active actions needed to navigate a crisis and providing credibility when future items need to be acted upon.

(3) **Leveraging opportunity in crisis**

A crisis can be a highly chaotic and disruptive event that leaves institutions, teams, and individuals with varying degrees of trauma [9]. Early on in the post-crisis phase, it is critical for a leader to conduct a rapid assessment of the existing landscape, analyzing all operational facets (administrative, clinical, financial) while remaining humble enough to recognize the lessons learned. How did we do? What did we do well? Where did we underperform? Asking these types of questions will guide the rebuilding process and help prepare the team for recovery and resumption. The progressive leader will then leverage this post-crisis assessment phase to identify opportunities where they can incorporate innovate strategies, since the instinct of "returning to normal" may not be the best philosophy in a post-crisis setting. These innovative opportunities can present in may forms, ranging from allocation of human capital to incorporating new systems and technologies. An example of this can been seen with the accelerated use of telemedicine technologies during the COVID crisis. Prior to March 2020, telemedicine was not mainstream in the American healthcare system, despite having the technological capabilities available for over a decade. However, the severity of the COVID pandemic necessitated the instantaneous shift toward delivering care virtually in a meaningful way. Institutional leaders began to incorporate video conferencing technologies that are built directly into their electronic medical record system to ensure a smooth user experience. Departmental leaders developed paradigms to systemically identify the types of visits appropriate for telemedicine to preserve access to care. The forward-thinking leader will take action on such opportunities, not only intra-crisis, but also sustainably, moving toward a "new normal."

Conclusion

Administrative leaders are tasked with creating an environment in which physicians, administrative staff and researchers can grow and prosper in their careers. This involves clinical practice efficiency, financial management, regulatory and billing compliance, effective marketing and outreach, educational program development, human resource management and talent acquisition, and creative scientific inquiry. The most effective administrative leaders take the time to be introspective to get clear about their motivations and leadership values. Additionally, there are several concrete strategies, some of which we touched on that can be helpful to employ as an aspiring clinical administrator, both during normal operations and times of crisis. With the ever-increasing demands on the time and effort of clinicians, taking on the role of an administrative leader may seem like yet another burden posed to today's urologist. However, it is our experience that when done well it can provide professional rewards unlike any other aspect of your career. In fact, Clayton may have summed these rewards when he said "Leadership is the most noble of professions if it's practiced well. Nothing else helps others learn and grow, take responsibility, and be recognized for their achievements." [10]. It is with this in mind that we encourage you to pursue your own administrative leadership journey and hope these principles may guide you along the way.

References

1. Thomason S. Becoming a physician executive: where to look before making the leap. 1999. https://www.aafp.org/fpm/1999/0700/p37.html. Accessed 9 Jan 2019.
2. Kornacki M. Three starting points for physician leadership. 2017. https://catalyst.nejm.org/three-starting-points-physician-leadership. Accessed 9 Jan 2019.
3. Harrington J, McNellis T. Mobilizing the right lean metrics for success. 2006. https://www.qualitydigest.com/may06/articles/02_article.shtml. Accessed 9 Jan 2019.
4. Welch K, Welch S. Winning. Harper Business Publishers. © 2005.
5. Drucker P. The essential Drucker. Collins Business Essentials. © 2008.
6. Bhimanprommachak V. Leading your team through a crisis. 2020 https://www.harvardbusiness.org/leading-your-team-through-a-crisis/. Assessed 27 Nov 2021.
7. Hoyt D. Looking forward. 2020. https://bulletin.facs.org/2020/07/looking-forward-july-2020/. Accessed 25 Nov 2021.
8. Kurtzman JT, Moran GW, Anderson CB, McKiernan JM. A novel and successful model for redeploying urologists to establish a closed intensive care unit within the emergency department during the COVID-19 crisis. J Urol. 2020;204(5):901–2.
9. Kaul V, Shah V, El-Serag H. Leadership during crisis: lessons and applications from the COVID-19 pandemic. Gastroenterology. 2020;159(3):809–12.
10. Christensen C. How will you measure your life?. 2010. https://hbr.org/2010/07/how-will-you-measure-your-life. Assessed 9 Jan 2019.

Chapter 7
The Urologist as Researcher

Wade Bushman

Research in Urology

Research in urology is characterized by enormous breadth, ranging from basic laboratory research to clinical trials and everything in between. These different avenues of investigation demand different levels of investment in money and time and need to be considered individually.

> Four Major Types of Urologic Research
> Bench Research
> Translational Research
> Health Services Research
> Clinical Research.

Bench Research is, quite simply, tough sledding. It requires high labor input and a lot of money. You simply cannot do it yourself and that means getting good help (no easy challenge) and managing people well. The difficulties inherent in this should not be underestimated. Nothing in medical education prepares us for managing people in the laboratory and, in general, the culture clash between MD's and Ph.D.'s can be a major stumbling block. For someone venturing into an independent laboratory research effort for the first time, an experienced mentor to provide not just scientific guidance, but advice in putting together a productive laboratory, is key. Finally, lab research is slow and time-consuming. You should figure on at least two to three years from starting project to paper submission.

W. Bushman (✉)
Department of Urology, University of Wisconsin School of Medicine and Public Health, Madison, WI, USA
e-mail: bushman@urology.wisc.edu

© The Author(s), under exclusive license to Springer Nature Switzerland AG 2022
S. Y. Nakada and S. R. Patel (eds.), *Navigating Organized Urology*,
https://doi.org/10.1007/978-3-031-05540-9_7

Translational research comes in a variety of flavors. For the sake of simplicity, we will focus on one example—application of basic science techniques to clinical specimens. This kind of research is most often collaborative—combining the efforts of basic scientists, clinicians, pathologists and/or biostatisticians. When compared to purely basic/bench research, this type is less labor intensive but still usually requires expertise and assistance beyond the senior investigators, such as lab personnel, residents or fellows. It is often moderately expensive, requiring money for specimen processing and pay-for-service analyses. An interval of one to two years from starting a project to paper submission would not be an unreasonable expectation.

Health Services Research is a rapidly expanding area. One great advantage of this kind of research is it's clear-cut relevance. Whether using existing or constructed databases to address issues of current importance in a timely way, develop new clinical protocols, or standardize practice methods, it can make a real impact over the short term. Costs are generally less than for bench or translational research and the interval from starting project to paper submission vary—but can be on the order of one to two years.

Clinical research embraces everything from a retrospective analysis of clinical data/practice/outcomes to prospective trial design. The labor input, requisite financial commitment and research infrastructure needs vary tremendously. For a simple retrospective chart review, it may be no more than six months from starting project to paper submission. For a prospective clinical trial, it may be up to five years.

Finding Your Niche

Individuals choose to pursue a research interest for a variety of reasons. What is yours?

Is it an expectation, and therefore, obligatory? Is it to gain recognition in your field?

Or to become a leader in your field? Is your primary motivation to help people? Is it to improve how things are done because you have a perfectionist bent? Or are you just insatiably curious and/or innovative? Answering this simple question honestly is critically important to getting onto the right path.

If doing research is to meet an expectation, then it can be a real drag. Do not shoot for the stars because of ego, you will be miserable. My advice is to find a relatively easy path that interests you and go for low hanging fruit. Just pick something doable and get it done. If your goal is recognition in your field, then focus your work in a specific area that is highly relevant to your area of practice and publish. If you want to be a leader in your field, focus your work in a specific area and publish often in top journals and speak whenever you have the chance. If your true motivation is a desire to help people, then identify areas of lagging progress or real unaddressed need. If you are channeling your perfectionist bent, focus on innovation in your clinical area. If it is the case that you are insatiably curious and/or innovative, then follow your passion(s) but avoid being diffuse. Try to work on topics relevant to your clinical field and crosslink your efforts so that they are self-reinforcing and amplifying.

Writing a Paper

Writing papers becomes easier with practice and repetition. But the important thing is to get started. Different people have different ways of doing it—but this works well for most people.

It is an approach the minimizes time spent trying to figure out what to say—leading naturally from the mechanical and objective to the narrative and speculative. These are the ordered steps:

Title Not the final title. But a title which succinctly states what you did and what it shows.

Materials and Methods Do this first. It is very mechanical and gets you into the writing groove.

Graphs and Tables This is the data that drives the paper. Think about how to put the data together and present it in a logical way that tells a logical story; it is the most important part of the paper and the part that takes the most thought. Once these are done, the results section will almost write itself.

Results Write as a simple narrative of what was done and what was found. Do not overthink it or exaggerate the findings—just the facts. Do not offer interpretations or speculations. If one observation led to another, state in very simple terms why that next step was made.

Plagiarism is bad but imitation is the greatest form of flattery. It is okay and extremely helpful to find a good paper in the similar area and/or of a similar nature and imitate the presentation of the data and results.

Discussion Briefly explain how your work addresses the question you are tackling. Summarize the results in a way that is not simply a reiteration of the results section but synthesizes the information and forms the basis for your conclusions; do not oversell. Reference previously done work in the area and describe how it complements, augments or extends previous studies. Point out the limitations of your study, unanswered questions and avenues for future work.

Introduction Write this dead last. Make it very simple. Define the problem or question addressed by your work. Set up the study—making that case as best you can that the study done was the best possible way to answer the question.

Presentation Skills

Presentation skills will improve with experience, but it is not the only way to improve. Read a book on the subject. Attend a workshop. Seek out an opportunity to see yourself recorded giving a talk or presentation. It is important to see how you come across—how others see you. It is said that 90% of what the audience takes away from any presentation is their impression of the speaker.

For any presentation, less is ALWAYS better. Scientific studies have shown that talks that go longer than scheduled are much more likely to be rated as boring. Too much information kills many a good talk. Keep it simple. A good tactic is to start by telling the audience what you're going to tell them. Then tell them. And end by telling them what you told them.

Finding Funding

The necessity of funding to support research varies with time commitment and the type of research to be done. A substantial time commitment to research often merits protected time. The goal of success in research needs to be a shared goal. For a clinician, the opportunity cost of protected time is quite significant. The faculty member should recognize this and understand that it cannot be an open-ended commitment and may require some concession in terms of expected salary. Most importantly, the amount and longevity of protected time should be negotiated at the time of recruitment. Depending on the nature of the position and research goals, some start-up funds may be provided by the department or the university.

Sources of Research Funding
Intramural research programs
American Urologic Association
Society grants
Corporate Funding
Veterans Administration
Department of Defense
National Institute of Health.

There are seven main sources of funding that can be pursued. The first is intramural research programs at your university. The second is the American Urologic Association (AUA). The third is societies such as the American Diabetes Association. The fourth is corporate support. The fifth is the Veterans Administration (VA). The last two are national funding sources such as Department of Defense (DOD) and the National Institute of Health (NIH).

Intramural Research Programs An example would be pilot funding opportunities through a comprehensive cancer center. Connect with the grants administration employees that work with your department and ask them for leads.

AUA The Research Scholar Award provides support for either one or two years for fellows and early career investigators. For a young clinician-scientist, this requires a 50%-time commitment to research. The award can also be used to support a basic scientist working under your supervision. The Summer Medical Student Fellowship can provide $4000 for support of a medical student during a 10-week mentored research experience. These awards are a great source of funding—but require thinking and advanced planning—so investigate them at your earliest opportunity.

Society Grants Cancer societies are pre-eminent in providing new investigator grants. It's slimmer pickings for benign urologic disease, but it pays to look in all the corners. The grants administration people can be of some help. Colleagues in the same field is another source of information. Also pay attention to acknowledgements of papers in your field, there are often specific funding opportunities for specific conditions such as interstitial cystitis and societies often maintain a list of relevant funding opportunities.

Corporate Funding Corporations have deep pockets and it can be tempting to pursue funding through a collaboration but beware of some pitfalls. First, the money rarely comes without strings attached. The company usually has its own agenda and your research focus may be distorted or mis-directed as a result of the collaboration. Secondly, beware of conflict of interest. This issue gets more complicated by the day and you should talk to the COI people at your institution before getting involved in anything that is supported by corporate funding. Finally, collaboration with a corporation on something like a clinical trial, even a simple one, can put financial liabilities on the department. It is important to allow the departmental administrator(s) vet the agreement to determine if there is potential for the department to be on the hook for a big chunk of money. The bottom line: corporate funding comes with a lot of potential pitfalls and it is important to talk to a lot of people, including your chair, departmental administrator, grants administrator and COI folks early on and heed their advice.

Veterans Administration The VA offers a variety of funding mechanisms; holding a VA research award requires a 5/8th commitment that can be split between clinical activities and research time. Importantly, this is a requirement for being awarded funding, but is not required to apply for funding. For someone seriously interested in pursuing research, the VA is arguably the most stable platform available for combing clinical work with investigative activities because the clinical obligations are generally well-defined and limited, the research time is paid out of the 5/8th appointment and the funds for research are comparable to an NIH R01.

Department of Defense (DOD) The DOD is best known for funding programs in prostate cancer and, more recently, kidney cancer. They publish annual program announcements that often include opportunities for new investigators. In addition, the DOD offers Career Development Awards in bladder cancer.

National Institute of Health (NIH) The NIH is made up of 27 different institutes and centers. The most significant for urologic research are the National Cancer Institute (NCI) and the National Institute of Diabetes and Digestive and Kidney Diseases (NIDDK). The NIDDK is the primary funding source of benign urologic disease research but other institutes, such as the National Institute on Aging also play a role. The NCI and NIDDK offer a variety of research awards. R01 is the primary individual investigator research award. These are highly competitive and require strong preliminary data. R21 is a pilot research funding mechanism that does not require preliminary data but is made stronger if it is included. The R21 is also quite competitive and is not available in all institutes. There are also funding mechanisms for multi-investigator initiatives, center grants and clinical studies. It is reasonable to say that NIH funding is really the province of the deeply committed investigator. The highly competitive nature of NIH funding has led to the development of Career Development (K) Awards to help young investigators become competitive for individual investigator awards. K awards can be obtained by application to the programs of the different institutes, K-programs awarded to and administered by NIH-funded clinical/translational research centers or K Scholar programs in Urologic Research awarded to a handful of Urology programs in the country. When it comes to looking into funding opportunities from the NIH there is one piece of advice commonly given and all too rarely taken: *Talk to your program officer*. All too often, the NIH is seen as a tight-fisted ogre that doesn't want to fund research. To the contrary, the NIH has as its highest priority the funding of the best scientific research proposals. The first step in achieving this goal is to help investigators identify the most suitable funding opportunities and to provide advice and direction in pursuing those opportunities. Talk to your research office and *then talk to your program officer at the institute to which you expect to apply*. They will welcome the opportunity to talk to you.

Grant Writing

A successful grant application requires *both* outstanding science *and* a superbly written proposal. Grant writing combines the art of persuasion with rigorous scientific thinking and is a skill that is challenging to learn and almost impossible to master. Even the most experienced and successful scientists have grants torn apart and rejected by a study section, so never underestimate the time, devotion and hard work required to be successful. It is a learning process and you should take advantage of any relevant learning opportunity. The AUA is offering both online and in-person grant writing workshops; seek them out. Find a mentor who is willing and able to put a lot of time helping you think critically about your research and critiquing your grantsmanship.

There are some absolute essentials for any grant effort. The first is to get an example of a successful application for whatever kind of proposal you plan to write, study it and use it as a model for your own proposal. The second is to follow the directions from the program announcement to the letter. If it says in the announcement to describe how the data will be acquired and stored—then you should have a small section that says exactly how the data will be collected and stored. Seriously. The third is to think about how much time it will take you to put together the proposal and realize that your estimate is way too optimistic. Most experienced grant writers will tell you that it takes them at least 9 months of hard work to produce a competitive proposal. Writing the proposal itself is relatively straightforward. It's thinking through the science, the planned studies, the analysis and the potential pitfalls and alternative strategies that takes the time. Many experienced grant writers say that it can take 6 months to come up with an abstract and specific aims that jumps off the page like the preview of a blockbuster movie. And, that is what it takes. If you haven't got the reviewers totally pumped by the time they finish reading your abstract, you will not get funded, it's really that simple.

Chung Lee, Ph.D. is a Professor Emeritus of Urology at Northwestern and an extremely accomplished grantsman. These are his rules for writing a successful grant application.

Rules for Writing a Successful Grant Application.
(Articulated by Dr. Chung Lee, Northwestern University).
All proposals must be hypothesis driven!
Come up with a hypothesis which is only one step ahead of the current state of knowledge—a statement that explains a mechanism in biology.
Rationale: Present a series of indirect observations that substantiate the above statement, including work done by others and your preliminary work.
Methods: Make a series of speculations and predictions of results, if the hypothesis is true, before describing what you want to do.
Make sure all methodologies are sound and thorough. Avoid descriptive studies.
Make disclaimers on issues that you cannot resolve before the reviewers catch them.
Point out the wonderful aspects of your study explicitly. Otherwise, they may not be appreciated.
In between sentences, show off your confidence, enthusiasm, honesty and novelty.

The Role of a Mentor

A young faculty member starting out in the world of research is a bit like a college kid painting the bedroom in his/her first apartment. The job will probably get done but it won't be pretty and won't be efficient. A good research mentor is like a professional painter who gives the kid advice: First spackle the holes and sand them smooth; then tape the molding, etc. Face it, you don't have all the time in the world (like a college kid does) to futz around. You need to be focused and efficient and nothing will help you achieve that like a seasoned mentor. A mentor does not have to have expertise in your specific area. Good, experienced mentors bring to the table a variety of skills that apply to a broad range of research. They will ask the hard questions that you need to face—upfront—before you go down an unproductive path. They will help you focus your interest; develop good, answerable research questions, push you to be self-critical and encourage you when you meet seemingly endless obstacles and disappointments. An exceptional mentor is one that makes your success a paramount consideration and does not seek any benefit or recognition from your work other than a thank you.

Time Management

Research takes time—a lot of time. Bench and translational research are usually tedious and time-intensive for the principal investigator. No matter where you are in your career—whether a new investigator or an old hand—the fact is that a lot of your research-related work will be done on nights and weekends. That is just a fact. All the rest of your—protected time, efficiency and any resources you can muster will never, ever change that. It will just make it possible for your work nights and weekends to put you "over the top."

Protected time is, generally, the province of the dedicated investigator—someone who plans to make research a centerpiece of their career. Protected time needs to be negotiated upfront. It may not need to be utilized immediately but a commitment from the department to support your research with protected research time when it is needed must be made before you start—or you will never get it. The reality is that most departments are feeling a financial squeeze and need to maximize clinical income. If your department's expectations do not allow for enough research time, then you have 3 options. Revise your guaranteed salary downward in exchange for research time, significantly revise your career plan, or consider another institution. The worst thing you can do for your career is to embark on a research plan with insufficient time and resources. You will fail.

You only get one shot at being a young faculty member with a guaranteed salary and some degree of protection from overwhelming clinical and administrative responsibilities. So, make it count. Talk with people and get a very clear idea of what you want your career and practice/research time commitments to look like in 7 years. You should plan out every one of the first seven years of your career with a timeline of expected accomplishments. Be specific and be realistic. Having a plan and a roadmap is essential. As noted by the immortal Yogi Bera: "If you don't know where you're going, you might not get there."

Work to make your clinic as efficient and productive as possible. The most important thing for the success of a talented clinician-scientist is to run your practice like a business. Mimic the most successful practitioners. Develop a referral base for remunerative procedures that you enjoy. Check your billings to make sure they are billing properly for what you do. And, focus on getting the most done in the least amount of time. Constantly work at being a profitable business and it will leave more time for scholarly activities.

Work to become more efficient. Look at the successful senior members of your department. You'll find they get more done in a week than would seem humanly possible. They do this by being incredibly efficient. They weren't born this way—they just worked at it over time. So should you. Do not get stuck in a slow, inefficient work habits. Think like an industrial engineer—find a better, faster way to do everything. Talk to your senior department members, learn their secrets and imitate them. In the end, it really is a foot-race. The more efficient you are the faster you can move and the more ground you can cover—and still be home in time for dinner.

Protect your own time. If you do not, it will get eaten away and you will get eaten alive. The clinical need is never-ending, and it is so easy to get pulled in. No one else is going to watch out for your time so you need to watch out for yourself. Obviously, patients always come first, and you never should say no to an unmet need. Many times, however, the attraction of being called on, of being needed and the good feeling that comes with making a difference entices a dereliction of your research activities. Do not let it happen. Decide up front how important research is to you and, if it is a priority, then be true to that priority. If with time you decide that your heart is in the clinic and the OR, then it is quite reasonable to amend the career plan, your priorities and your time commitments.

Leading a Research Team

Most research efforts require collaboration and a team. It often is the case that interpersonal skills are as important as scientific acumen in achieving progress toward goals of the research.

Recruitment of people to assist in the research is a critical step and knowing what you can and cannot reasonably expect of those you recruit is critical. A common example of mismatch between expectations and skills is the physician who wants to "hire a Ph.D." to run their research program and/or their lab. A well-trained degree scientist brings to the table honed skills in performing research, addressing scientific questions with well-designed and well-controlled studies subject to rigorous analysis and interpretation. The doctoral degree does not prepare anyone to oversee a research program, mentor others or ensure compliance with all the regulatory rules governing research in the current era. The principal investigator (PI) has ultimate responsibility for all of these and while some elements may be delegated with careful oversight, the weight of it will always fall squarely on the PI. The take-home message is that people should not be recruited into the research effort with the expectation that they will take something off the PI's plate, but rather, that they leverage the PI's efforts to more efficiently achieve goals of the research.

Recruiting the right people is key. Doing so is a combination of good judgment and good luck. Luck brings the right people to you; judgment allows you to make the right choice. It is tempting to pick someone with "experience" because it would seem to make it easier and faster to get off the ground, but in the long run aptitude and personal qualities are more critical. To put it in concrete terms, in looking for a lab tech, I would pass up a person who got a 3.5 in the sciences and worked for two years in a lab after college but didn't really get along all that will the PI, for new grad who was a successful athlete in high school, balanced academic achievement with part-time work in college and got a 3.9 in history with just a couple of science courses. The first has experience. The second has potential.

A rule that has always served well is to be as forthright and transparent as possible. The only hiring situation that reliably works out well is where everyone involved makes a well-informed decision that is in their best interest. You should never hire someone because you feel sorry for them or because you think you can change their trajectory. Likewise, you should never sell anyone on a position that really isn't in their best interest. Play it straight.

You can never expect anyone else to care about the research as much as you. Face it: most people don't live to work. For them it's a job, not a passion. And they don't owe you any favors. The key is to identify what motivates each person with whom you work and figure out how to make working with you meet those wants and needs. Strive to make every person you work with successful in their own eyes. Do that, and they will follow you and make you proud.

Empower every person you work with. Divest your "ownership" of the research and make all the other contributors the stakeholder. Don't ever make the mistake of thinking that people work for you. Make it clear that they work for themselves. In a football analogy, be the coach not the team owner. Spend time and energy being a coach for every person in your group to help them in life—not just in your research efforts. Know their situation. Their family. Their troubles.

Encourage teamwork. Model hard work and teamwork. But don't shy away from hard decisions in people management. If someone isn't being a team-player, address it. As an aside—surgeons are often less than ideal team players. They are used to people getting them whatever they want when they need it, getting everything ready for them and cleaning up after them. If you have physicians as part of your group, be alert for the ripples they will cause.

Half the people in the world are below average, and even those that are above average are off their game some of the time. Everybody makes mistakes. Respect that people are trying their best, even when they fail in spectacular fashion. It's ok and necessary to offer constructive criticism of methods, performance etc.—but always with encouragement. Be extremely careful to not embarrass or humiliate, even unconsciously. A little self-deprecating humor can defuse what for a junior person can be an extremely emotional moment. Never let your temper get the best of you and never fire off an angry email. A good rule of thumb is that any significant criticisms or frank talk should be done in private and after the heat of the moment has passed.

Success in research comes more frequently than unicorn sightings, but not much. When it does, it's essential that the credit goes to everyone else. It is *their* research efforts, *their* work, *their* success. You can take pride in having built the team that achieved that success.

Chapter 8
Academic Roles: Inventor

Ryan L. Steinberg, Brett A. Johnson, and Jeffrey A. Cadeddu

Introduction

Academic urologists must balance a multitude of roles as part of their work, including but not limited to clinician, partner, educator, researcher, and mentor. In fulfilling these roles, many will identify a need for new technology or areas of improvement for existing technology. For the motivated urologist, this provides the groundwork to pursue the development of new devices or improve currently available technology. Furthermore, as many academic medical centers are often associated with a university or undergraduate/graduate college, the ability to cultivate collaborative relationships with others (e.g. engineers, scientists, and business) may help drive these pursuits. In this chapter, we aim to highlight the process to inventorship and share thoughts, advice and common pitfalls of the process.

Identify the Need

The fundamental notion of any invention is first identifying a need for the product. In some cases, this is straightforward. For example, people who previously underwent transurethral resection of the prostate (TURP) using monopolar loop cautery were at risk of developing TURP syndrome (hyponatremia) due to intravascular absorption of free water. The need was clear: avoid a common and possibly fatal complication of surgery. The bipolar resectoscope was thus developed, which utilized saline in place of water, negating the possibility of TURP

R. L. Steinberg
Department of Urology, University of Iowa Hospitals and Clinics, Iowa City, IA, USA

B. A. Johnson · J. A. Cadeddu (✉)
Department of Urology, University of Texas Southwestern, Dallas, TX, USA
e-mail: jeffrey.cadeddu@utsouthwestern.edu

© The Author(s), under exclusive license to Springer Nature Switzerland AG 2022
S. Y. Nakada and S. R. Patel (eds.), *Navigating Organized Urology*,
https://doi.org/10.1007/978-3-031-05540-9_8

syndrome. While this is rather obvious, not all inventions must be so. Improvements in surgical equipment ergonomics, measurement methodology, and others can have large impacts on those who use the products. Furthermore, not all inventions require the creation of a physical object. Advances in computer programming and artificial intelligence are leading to a vast new array of software spanning a multitude of areas including automated cancer detection and structured feedback for surgical training. Identifying the need is the first step.

There are many obstacles in pursuit of advancement due to one of a number of factors, including time, financial ability, or the belief that others are already addressing this need. In a TEDx talk entitled "A tool to fix one of the most dangerous moments in surgery," Nikolai Begg, a biomedical engineering graduate student, discussed his design for the Veress needle to make insufflating the abdomen at the beginning of laparoscopic surgeries safer [1]. Begg negates the assumption that all major problems are actively being addressed by a panel of experts, urges those with an idea to allow the problem to captivate them, and encourages the pursuit of a solution with great zeal. He could not be more correct.

Invention Conceptualization

After identifying the need, possible solutions must be considered. This can be one of, if not the, most difficult aspects of inventorship, as it sets the stage for all other progress. Sometimes, simple modifications to existing products can drastically improve their function. Other times, a fundamentally new ideology is needed. Before beginning an endeavor to re-invent the wheel, a thorough search of what is commercially available can help to identify what has already been produced (occasionally, devices/equipment may be available but not purchased by the institution) and may spur ideas for new or re-designed devices. Likewise, it is possible that a new device has been developed but not brought to market due to an unforeseen obstacle. Next, an internet-based patent search and review of the available literature via PubMed, Google Scholar, and other such websites should be undertaken. It is during this step that collaboration may be particularly beneficial as existing protected products may exist in other fields not always reviewed by a new inventor.

After familiarizing yourself with what has already been investigated and reported, a written list considering all means to accomplishing your goal should be created. It is imperative to exclude no idea, even if you don't think it will work. In creating this exhaustive list, a review (or rapid education) in certain scientific principles/technologies may be required. For example, when considering measuring liquid flow, there are many a multitude of ways to do so, including mechanical (e.g. turbine rotations), pressure-based (e.g. pitot tube), optical-based (e.g. optical flow meter), imaging-based (e.g. sonar flow meter), etc. In the case of novel software, various programming languages, operating system/hardware compatibility, etc. should be considered. After creating the list, a critical appraisal of the constraints of the need (e.g. size/dimensions/compatibility) will often eliminate some of the ideas generated. The inventor will then need to select a concept with which to model or pursue for prototype production. While cost is typically not a significant concern when prototyping, some forethought should be given to marketability and scalability for a potential product.

Depending on the institution and desires of the academic urologist, inclusion of graduate students, engineering professors, medical students, residents, and fellows in the process of conceptualization can be incredibly helpful. Many of these individuals will have prior life experiences (e.g. college degrees in engineering, working in industry, knowledge of regulatory processes) that can be beneficial. Involvement in these types of activities can also be exciting for the trainee, as well as beneficial to his/her resume and spurn an interest in urology and/or device development.

Modeling

When considering computer modeling, it is important to distinguish between the use of this term in reference to a virtual design or a simulation in which the design is manipulated. Computer-aided design (CAD) can improve the accuracy (reduce human error) in developing plans for a prototype, as well as facilitate faster design modifications. There are now a multitude of software options to generate CAD drawings with one of the most recognized being AutoCAD® (San Rafael, CA, USA). Depending on the means of manufacturing (e.g. 3D printed parts, etc.), CAD may also be advantageous in preparation for computer-assisted manufacturing (CAM). Though, limitations of CAD include the cost of the software (though there are free tools available) and cost (both time and monetary) to learn how to use the software.

Computer simulation aims to create variations in the environment or on the virtual design itself. This allows engineers to better understand failure methods of the device. Computer simulation has shown the ability to expedite testing (e.g. failure testing), reduce costs, and avoid unethical experiments. Medical device evaluation historically has included laboratory, animal and human data. As of 2015, the Food and Drug Administration (FDA) noted a desire not for more total data with the inclusion of computer simulation data but the use of these data to create less reliance on animal and human data [2]. Since that time, the FDA has issued a guidance statement on reporting of computational modeling studies [3]. With the advances in computer simulation now possible, some inventors advocate the use of early computer simulation to aid in prototype development (e.g. guide material selection based on simulated device stress/strain evaluation). The decision to proceed with early simulation is inventor-dependent and project-specific.

Prototype

Prototyping is one of the more complex aspects of device development and requires expertise typically outside the realm of the urologist. This process has historically required the expertise of a broad range of engineering fields including mechanical, electrical, materials science, biomedical, supply chain, and computer science. Though, the landscape of prototyping has changed drastically over the past decade with several new and readily available technologies.

First, the advent of inexpensive three-dimensional (3D) printing (a microwave sized machine can cost only a few hundred dollars), which can utilize several different filament materials (raw materials) with unique properties to create parts of a device, has allowed for the rapid and low-cost prototype creation. The National Institute of Health (NIH) has a repository of biomedical CAD files available for free (https://3dprint.nih.gov/). Other advances include inexpensive ($\sim$ $20–$40), yet robust system-on-a-chip computers (e.g. Raspberry Pi (Raspberry Pi Foundation, Cambridge United Kingdom) and Arduino (open source)), which can be programmed, modified, and updated with ease to perform computation, sensor input/output, or electronic actuation. Further, simplified, user-friendly software to assist in CAD, 3D printing, and single-board computers has made these processes accessible to those without expertise in computer programming.

The typical prototyping process starts with a Proof-of-Concept (PoC) device. The PoC serves to verify the key functional aspects of the device without effort given to ease-of-use or aesthetics. PoCs are often "over-engineered," meaning that more versatile materials are used, which allow testing to be done at various levels of sensitivity and complexity. If the device works well with less precision, less costly components can be used for the massed produced product. In the case of software, an initial code is written and debugged, as well as a rudimentary user interface is developed to confirm device functionality.

Next, a Working Prototype (WP) is produced that uses similar engineering/technology and replicated all functionality as would be incorporated into a final device. Typically, the WP is used to test the device in a clinical environment and allow further technical refinements based on experimentation results. This is often where re-coding and further debugging to improve the efficiency of data processing is required for software, in addition to enhancing the user interface to optimize user satisfaction and efficiency of device use. A Visual Prototype (or "Mock-up") resembles the dimensions, appearance, and aesthetics of the final product and would follow a WP. The final stage before mass production is a Functional Prototype. This is essentially the final product and represents the appearance and function of the market-ready production device.

Testing

Device testing is critical for several reasons. Initially, the Proof-of-Concept prototype must demonstrate that the science and engineering behind the device work. Additional investigation establishes safety, reliability and reproducibility and the device. Ultimately, scientifically rigorous studies are needed to establish that the device is superior to (or at least equivalent to) the current standard of care. Additionally, testing is done to determine the precision required for the components of the device. Typically, stricter tolerance for component variance comes at significant cost of manufacturing. It is critical to determine how to reduce cost and improve scalability while maintaining integrity of the device. This allows the device to be mass-produced at a reasonable unit cost.

As it would be unethical to directly use novel devices on patients, prototypes must first establish safety and efficacy in a study model. Models come in different forms and are made to suit the stage of development. Initial testing is often performed in vitro (in the lab) with simple materials with tissue-mimicking properties. Silicone, basic organic material (e.g. fruits or vegetables), and more advanced, 3D printed biomimetic materials can all be used to simulate tissues. For software, this would be an opportunity to test the program on small, constructed data sets. The goal of initial testing is to demonstrate device safety and reliability and often requires several design modifications to be made.

Later stages of development require more sophisticated models. Deceased animal organs (e.g. porcine or bovine kidneys and bladders) can often be obtained for relatively low cost and without the need of prior approval in the case of physical equipment. Likewise, the cadaveric model is a critical tool for testing and development of medical devices. Fresh tissue cadavers offer an excellent anatomical model while not requiring Institutional Review Board (IRB) approval. The drawback is the cost of the model and can range from several hundred to a few thousand dollars depending on the location, institution, and tissue needs. It is at this stage that software would be trialed on a large scale of real-world data to confirm accuracy and reliability.

In vivo testing is often initially accomplished with living animal models. Small mammal, canine, or porcine models tend to be the most commonly used. Mammalian models often require approval from Institutional Animal Care and Use Committee (IACUC). Protocols involving animal testing have to be well designed and well described before starting any testing. While renal anatomy is well modeled in the animal model, canine and porcine urethras are not similar to humans and often present a challenge to models that require transurethral access.

The final stage of testing requires human subjects. Protocols involving patients or healthy volunteers require strict approval by the IRB, require patient consent, and registration of the study with ClinicalTrials.gov. In some cases of negligible risk of harm, informed consent can be waived. Rigorous testing protocols should be designed to compare the device against the standard of care. The designer of the protocol must give thought to powering the study appropriately, proper randomization, and an appropriate control. The goal of the investigation is to determine device safety (Phase I), work consistently across different testing environments (Phase II), and determine how the device compares to current standard of care (Phase III).

Funding

The process of designing, prototyping, and testing a novel device can be incredibly expensive. Funding such projects is critical to their success. The United States spent approximately $450 billion on research and development in 2013, 71% of which came from the private sector [4]. The source of research funding can be broken down into public or private funds. The National Institutes of Health (NIH) is the largest public funder of biomedical research in the world. The NIH awards grant to fund medical research according to a peer-reviewed process. There are several types of awards. The most common is an R01, which is used to support a discrete, specified, research project. A K-award is designed for career development of scientists early in their career. Congressional appropriation for the NIH has decreased in the past decade and R01-equivalent grants are extremely competitive. In general, NIH grants are not used to commercialize product, but rather contribute to the body of science in the community.

An additional source of public funding that is often a better approach to medical device funding than an R01 is a Small Business Innovation Research (SBIR) grant. These awards are intended to help small businesses conduct research and development. These grants seek to contribute to the development of a specific product with potential for commercialization. The SBIR grant was created to fund early-stage innovation for possibly industry-changing ideas that are too high-risk for private investors. The SBIR programs are tiered with the first phase awarding $150,000 for initial exploration of feasibility. More information can be found at www.SBIR.gov.

Private funding sources can likewise be used to support the development of medical research. Some academic institutions have endowments to support certain types of research. Private funding for researchers also can also come from philanthropists, crowd-funding, private medical or device companies, non-profit foundations, or professional organizations like the American Urology Association. Declaring the source of funding as well as any possible conflicts of interest is critical in the process of scientific discovery.

Intellectual Property Protection

One of the most important aspects of inventorship is the protection of intellectual property. This point cannot be understated. The easiest way to begin protecting your property is to keep a timestamped (date and time) paper trail (be it actual paper or electronic documents/art), regardless of the simplicity, poor grammar, or bad artistic skills. We recommend keeping a bound journal or notebook to record ideas, thoughts, schematics, technical drawings, and anything related to your idea/invention. Some recommend numbering the pages sequentially, not skipping pages, initialing the entries, and having witnesses to your records. These added steps can confirm the validity of your documentation but also can be laborious. These records of your developmental process are a great way to stay organized and in the case of a dispute regarding the legal inventor, can provide proof of the invention date.

The United States Patent and Trademark Office (USPTO) offers multiple types of protections including trademark, copyright, service mark, and patent within the United States only. The definition of each is specified in Table 8.1. It is important to appreciate the differences between these options to ensure that you are obtaining the correct protection. With inventorship, most will ultimately decide to pursue a patent, specifically a utility patent. Though, patents can be difficult to obtain when attempting to protect software. In such circumstances, a copyright may be the most advantageous route of protection as it can protect the source code and unique elements of a user interface. It is also important to understand that a separate international patent must be applied for if protections are to extend to countries outside of the US. It should be stressed that the available options offer protection of an invention, not simply an idea. In most circumstances, an idea will evolve into sufficient detail regarding how to accomplish the desired endpoint (fulfilling the

Table 8.1 Definitions of common types of protections offered by the US patent and trademark office

Types of protection	Definition
Trademark	A word, phrase, symbol, and/or design that identifies and distinguishes the source of the goods of one party from those of others
Service mark	A word, phrase, symbol, and/or design that identifies and distinguishes the source of a service rather than goods. Some examples include: brand names, slogans, and logos
Patent	A limited duration property right relating to an invention, granted by the United States Patent and Trademark Office in exchange for public disclosure of the invention. Patentable materials include machines, manufactured articles, industrial processes, and chemical compositions
Copyright	Protects original works of authorship including literary, dramatic, musical, and artistic works, such as poetry, novels, movies, songs, computer software, and architecture

Source   https://www.uspto.gov/trademarks-getting-started/trademark-basics/trademark-patent-or-copyright

previously identified need), which would constitute an invention [5]. It is important to consider this prior to pursuing a patent.

Prior to filing a patent, there are a few important considerations. First and foremost: Is the idea mine? Gattari provides a thorough list on whom would not be considered an inventor, including someone who contributes to the device but only an obvious element [5]. After confirming that the idea is your own, a thorough patent search should be undertaken as patent applications can cost $5,000–$10,000 excluding patent attorney fees. This can be performed online either on the USPTO website, a patent database site, or Google Patents. A common pitfall is to assume that if the device/product is not on the market then it is not patented. It is not uncommon for devices to be patented but never come to market. This can be as a result of difficulties during testing, obtaining FDA approval or purchasing of patents by companies to limit market competition.

When pursuing patent protection, inventors have two choices. They can file for a provisional patent application or a full patent. A provisional application allows an inventor to establish an earlier official filing date for a patent, assuming that a full patent application is submitted. A provisional application has a life of 1 year. If a full patent is not filed at the end of a provisional application, the early filing date is negated. Thus, if a full patent is to be pursued, a provisional application can help provide a year of protection to continue development and perform testing in support of a full patent application. A fully executed utility patent has a life of 15 years from the date of issuance. As of May 2021, the average time from utility patent application filing to final disposition (patent issued or abandonment) is currently estimated to be 22.9 months with a backlog of 619,219 unexamined applications [6]. During this time, amendments can be made to the application; therefore, it is critical to continue development and testing during this time. The added data can only strengthen an application.

In your patent application, the goal of the invention claims is to demonstrate that your device is useful, novel, and non-obvious. These are critical words to consider when filing as each needs to be fulfilled for a patent to be issued. The USPTO offers an 'Inventors Assistance Center' through the www.uspto.gov website which can be helpful in assessing if your device meets these criteria. Though, in our experience, a knowledgeable patent attorney can be extremely helpful in these circumstances.

A common question that is asked is when an inventor should approach industry with their idea/invention. While a well-documented notebook provides the time of idea inception and development, we advise a conservative strategy when discussing any ideas or devices with industry. We suggest some form of patent application be filed prior to any meeting in which intellectual property will be discussed. We caution inventors about opening dialogue with industry under a provisional application unless the filing of a full patent is a guarantee given that the advanced filing date protection will lapse after only 1 year.

FDA Approval

The Food and Drug Administration, a federal agency within the United States Department of Health and Human Services, is responsible for the protection of public health by overseeing the production of pharmaceutical drugs and medical devices (among other things). Not all devices require approval by the FDA, but for those that do, there are two regulatory pathways. The far most common is the 510 (k) process. In this pathway the manufacturer submits a Premarket Notification to the FDA to demonstrate the device is as safe and effective as an existing FDA-approved device on the market. The other pathway is Premarket Approval (PMA), and it is much more rigorous than 510(k) pathway and is for devices that do not have a comparable device already on the market. The device manufacturer submits information about how the device is designed and manufactured as well as clinical trials demonstrating its safety and efficacy. The 510(k) process is much more cost-effective and 99% of new devices use this pathway.

The FDA classifies medical devices into three categories. A Class I device has low to moderate risk to the patient. About half of all medical devices fall within this category. Most devices in this category are exempt from regulation and premarket notification or approval is not required. The manufacturer is required to register with the FDA and report any adverse outcomes. Examples of Class 1 devices are examination gloves, bandages, basic surgical instruments. A Class II device has moderate to high risk to the patient. These devices (with a few exceptions) require Premarket Notification or Approval as well as post-market surveillance. These devices are held to a higher level of assurance than Class I devise. Examples of Class II devices include surgical drapes, infusion pumps, ureteral stents, and ureteroscopes. Class III devices either have significant risk or there is insufficient information to accurately determine risk. These devices require Premarket Approval and extensive pre-market investigation. Examples of such devise are implantable devices, defibrillators, HIV tests, and ureteral bulking agents. Most new devices fall within the first two classes and follow the 510(k) processes.

When studying a novel medical device prior to any pre-market action with the FDA, an investigational device exemption (IDE) allows the device to be used in clinical study with the goal of collecting safety and effectiveness data. Unless the device is exempt from pre-market approval, devices must seek an IDE prior to study. The study must be approved by the local IRB, and if there is significant risk to patients, the FDA must also review the investigation plan. Informed consent, proper labeling (investigational use only) and close monitoring is required for an IDE to be approved. More information can be found at: https://www.fda.gov/MedicalDevices/.

Key Points:

- Identify where there is a need and consider ways to address the problem.
- Keep a log of ideas/developments and limit discussion early on to help protect your ideas.
- Prototyping has become more rapidly and less costly than in years past due to new technologies.
- Start testing on simple models (in vitro) and proceed to more complex ones if results appear promising.
- Multi-disciplinary collaboration is often a critical component of achieving success when developing a device.

Compliance with Ethical Requirement Ryan L. Steinberg, Brett A. Johnson, and Jeffrey A. Cadeddu declare that they have no conflict of interest.

References

1. Begg N. A tool to fix one of the most dangerous moments in surgery. TEDx Beacon Street 2013. p. https://www.ted.com/talks/nikolai_begg_a_tool_to_fix_one_of_the_most_dangerous_moments_in_surgery.
2. Morrison TM. Using Modeling and Simulation for Medical Device Innovation: Virtual Patients for Regulatory Decision Making. 2015 FDA Science Writers Symposium 2015.
3. Center for Devices and Radiological Health: Office of Device Evaluation. Reporting of Computational Modeling Studies in Meidcal Device Submissions: Guidance for Industry and Food and Drug Administration Staff. Deparmtnet of Health and Human Services 2016.
4. Anonymous. Microbiology Policy Bulletin Board. Microbe Magazine. 2016;11(145).
5. Gattari PG. Determining inventorship for US patent applications. Intellectual Property and Technology Law Journal. 2005;17(5):16–9.
6. United States Patent and Trademark Office. USPTO Data Visualization Center: USPTO; 2018. Available from: https://www.uspto.gov/dashboards/patents/main.dashxml.

Chapter 9
Academic Research Collaboration

Kristina L. Penniston

Introduction

Year after year science provides more answers to problems, some of which were not even imagined a short time ago. Yet these answers raise an ever-increasing number of new questions. The more we know, it seems the more there is to know. The considerable gains in science and health knowledge in recent decades have given way in the twenty-first century to larger and more complex questions and new fields of inquiry: quantum biology, synthetic biology, microbiomics, genomics, metabolomics, nutrigenomics, exposomics, and so on. New approaches to health and biomedical science—"big data," population health, translational science, artificial intelligence, machine learning—have emerged. As basic scientists and clinician scientists delve ever deeper in an effort to answer these questions, and with higher demand for research findings to flow more quickly into clinical and community settings (translational science), investigators are increasingly driven to join together to share resources and pool their unique interdisciplinary expertise [1], taking the form of intra- and extramural as well as intra- and inter-institutional collaborations. Opportunities promoted by large funding agencies reflect this higher complexity of scientific inquiry and are driving the move toward scientific collaboration and "team science" [2, 3]. While the uptake of collaborative, interdisciplinary team science is variable, the interdisciplinarity of teams in the biomedical research sphere is increasingly linked with success with respect to scientific discovery, disruption, and impact. A recent review of the Thomson Reuters Web of Science database

K. L. Penniston (✉)
University of Wisconsin School of Medicine and Public Health, Department of Urology, Madison, WI 53705-2281, USA
e-mail: penn@urology.wisc.edu

UW Health University Hospital and Clinics, Department of Clinical Nutrition Services, 1685 Highland Avenue, 3258 Medical Foundation Centennial Building, Madison, WI 53705-2281, USA

revealed that the measure of research interdisciplinarity was significantly correlated with journal impact factor [4].

The number of multiple principal investigator (PI) grants funded by the National Institutes of Health (NIH) has risen over time, growing from only 3 in 2006 (its first year of multiple-PI grants) to 1,098 in 2013 [3]. Within the National Institute of Diabetes and Digestive Kidney Diseases (NIDDK), the growth in multiple PI awards in the R01/R37 portfolio increased from 6% in 2011 to 22% in 2020 [5]. In addition to the traditional R01 funding mechanisms, institutes across the NIH now offer an ever-growing number of program project and cooperative agreement grant opportunities; the percentage of funding for which these types of awards account has risen. For example, initially funded in 1994 through a grant mechanism, the multi-center Breast Cancer Surveillance Consortium is now a program project grant that received $17 million in a 2017 renewal award from the National Cancer Institute. The National Science Foundation (NSF) and other federal funding agencies have an even longer history of collaborative science models [3, 6]. The NSF began funding program grants >20 years earlier than did the NIH. While beginning with just one in 1985, in 2011 the NSF invested nearly $300 million in multiple center programs [6].

But while collaborative science is increasingly the norm and frequently a successful strategy for new scientific discovery, few of us are trained to engage in such research teams. Successful research collaborations do not just form on their own, nor do they succeed without the use of proven techniques and approaches. Moreover, impediments to engaging in collaborative research teams are not insignificant and include the lack of recognition in academic hiring practices [7] and in achieving tenure [8]. The purpose of this chapter is to: (1) provide a context and rationale for academic research collaborations; (2) identify critical features of successful collaborators and collaborations; (3) highlight some of the benefits and challenges of collaboration; and (4) share key lessons learned and "best practices" from my own experiences as a collaborator in both the clinical and research settings and as the director of the NIDDK-funded Urology Centers Program Interactions Core (U24-DK-127726).

Definitions, Rationale, and Features of Academic Collaboration

Definitions of collaboration. Merriam-Webster defines collaboration generally as "working jointly with others or together especially in an intellectual endeavor." There are many definitions that specifically describe academic collaborations (Table 9.1). Most interject some unique thought or aspect of collaboration. But there are common themes, including shared learning, endeavoring to create new knowledge (i.e., knowledge that would not be gained without the collaboration), complementary skills and expertise, coordinated resources, and shared responsibility. As collaborations develop across numerous disciplines, including biological

Table 9.1 Definitions of collaboration. The term "collaboration" has multiple meanings. The table lists several definitions for "collaboration" consistent with academic research and/or clinical cooperative relationships that are centered around common goals and mission

First author	Definitions
Denbo [9]	A means to producing knowledge that would otherwise never happen; sharing ideas with someone who focuses on another aspect of a subject, who knows related literature better, or who has expertise in another domain of knowledge altogether, enabling work that would otherwise be impossible
Schöttle [10]	Inter-organizational relationship with a common vision to create a common project organization with a commonly defined structure and a new and jointly developed project culture, based on trust and transparency; with the goal to jointly solve problems mutually through interactive processes, which are planned together, and by sharing responsibilities, risk, and rewards among the key participants
Bozeman [11]	Social processes whereby human beings pool their human capital for the objective of producing knowledge; a bringing together of talents for the purpose of knowledge creation and usually resulting in an identifiable knowledge product (e.g., scientific paper, patent, improved base of knowledge, enhanced academic reputation)
Bennett and Gadlin [7]	A group that is led by one or more scientists and is composed of researchers with diverse backgrounds and different areas of expertise and in which the collaborators will have developed common objectives, coordinated their resources, and composed a shared agenda of activities directed toward achieving those objectives
Baldwin and Chang and Bronstein [12, 13]	An effective interpersonal process that facilitates the achievement of goals that cannot be reached when individual professionals act on their own, the rationale for which includes: increasing prestige or influence; sharing resources and reducing costs; and/or facilitating learning
Dillenbourg [14]	A situation in which two or more people learn or attempt to learn something together; joint problem solving
Hardin [15]	The process of shared creation: two or more individuals with complementary skills interacting to create a shared understanding that none had previously possessed or could have come to on their own. Collaboration creates a shared meaning about a process, a product, or an event
Macrina [16]	Diverse partnerships between intra- or extramural investigative entities that are formed when researchers wish to take their research programs in new directions with goals of advancing knowledge enriching processes, and developing new products and outcomes
Roschelle and Teasley [17]	Coordinated, synchronous activity that is the result of a continued attempt to construct and maintain a shared conception of a problem; the mutual engagement of participants in a coordinated effort to solve a problem together

(continued)

Table 9.1 (continued)

First author	Definitions
Mattessich and Monsey [18]	A process that brings previously separated organizations (or individuals) into a new structure with full commitment to a common mission
Wood and Gray [19]	Collaboration occurs when a group of autonomous stakeholders of a problem domain engage in an interactive process, using shared rules, norms, and structures, to act or decide on issues related to that domain
Appley and Winder [20]	A relational system in which (1) individuals in a group share mutual aspirations and a common conceptual framework; (2) the interactions among individuals are characterized by "justice and fairness;" and (3) these aspirations and conceptualizations are characterized by each individual's consciousness of his/her motives toward the other; by caring or concern for the other; and by commitment to work with the other over time provided that this commitment is a matter of choice
Meadows [21]	Collaboration is a concrete form of readily observable networking wherein researchers work together on research project—designing it and/or undertaking the project together and publishing its results—to influence research funding and/or performance systems

science, social science, environmental science, physical science, and medical science, it makes sense that each is defined according to its unique needs and context. Some collaborations may work best when collaborators are equal partners pursuing mutually interesting and beneficial research. But collaborations may also involve researchers of differing stature, funding status, and types of organizations. As each collaboration involves different collaborators and serves a unique purpose, each is uniquely assembled and defined.

Research collaborations take different forms. They may be predominantly intradisciplinary (within one field or discipline), cross disciplinary, multidisciplinary, interdisciplinary, or transdisciplinary. There is no one definition for each of these. Although from a social science research perspective, Marilyn Stember offered definitions for each [22] that make sense for biomedical research. While intradisciplinary refers to research involving investigators from within a single field or discipline, cross disciplinary is research "viewing one discipline from the perspective of another" [22]. According to this definition, using the methods of one discipline to investigate and describe another would be an example (e.g., a bioinformatician using high throughput computer analysis techniques to study the microbiome). A more modern definition of cross disciplinary, and perhaps one more suited to biomedical research, is from Miller and Leffert [23], who described it as research that "synthesizes expertise from diverse contributing disciplines and develops new scientific approaches to address complex problems in health." Multidisciplinary research is uniformly considered "higher level" collaborative work that involves investigators from several disciplines, each providing their independent perspectives on a problem and contributing their individually-produced results to the final output or product. Toward the further end of the collaborative spectrum are interdependent research collaborations, which typically require a longer "incubation" period wherein investigators from different disciplines spend a significant amount of time exchanging and integrating knowledge resulting in shared perspective, mission, and goals. "Interdisciplinary" and "transdisciplinary" are monikers for these types of collaborations. Stember described interdisciplinary integration as the bringing together of the different parts of knowledge into "harmonious relationships" wherein investigators "take into account the contributions of others in making their own contributions" [22]. At the most collaborative end of the spectrum is transdisciplinary collaboration, requiring a higher level of immersion and unity that achieves interdependence through the development of a shared intellectual and conceptual framework that would not be possible in any other type of collaboration. An example might be a collaboration between a bioinformatics expert, a microbiologist, and a clinician-scientist to investigate the urinary microbiota and creating a new unified approach for further studies that encompasses the tools and knowledge from each discipline.

Rationale for collaboration. Scientific collaboration has long been promoted. In 1969, Donald T. Campbell, a social scientist and early proponent of a collaborative method of public policy that would use interdisciplinary experimentation and data as a guide for decision-making, proposed a collaborative model for research. Specifically, he suggested that science is most effective when researchers with expert knowledge in different areas collaborate on a project of overlapping interest [24]. Overlap allows for common ground, he reasoned, while the respective areas of expertise cover a greater "surface area" of the possible knowledge brought to bear on a specific question [25]. As scientific research has become more complex, universities and other research organizations have created innovative infrastructure to promote interactions, including open laboratory spaces, shared "core" equipment and resources, and public "interactions" areas [26]. Collaborative science increasingly transcends university boundaries. Indeed, in recent years, multi-university collaborations have been the fastest-growing type of authorship structure [27].

Not all science requires collaboration. But, given the increasing complexity of the health care system and patient conditions, and given the more specialized knowledge and resources required in biomedical and translational research that aims to understand and manage them, collaboration is appropriate. In their "field guide" to collaboration and "team science," Bennett et al. note the increasing "complexity of today's most pressing health issues and diseases" as requiring collaborations among scientists trained in different research methods [28]. The case highlighted in the **sidebar** offers a good example of how, when a particular research problem, aim, or mission is substantial and large enough to be subdivided into different research directions, collaboration allows for these different directions to be pursued and then tied together to form a broader yet cohesive picture of the problem.

Translational Collaboration in Urinary Stone Disease

Decades of research in urinary calcium oxalate stone disease have led to the widespread consensus that it is even more complex that many previously believed, with multiple etiologic factors and variably expression between affected individuals. In many ways, there are now more questions about calcium oxalate stone formation and growth than ever before.

New collaborative efforts to better understand how calcium oxalate stones grow—involving nephrologists and urologists as well as geological scientists and molecular biologists—have revealed novel insights about the crystalline architecture and chemistry of calcium oxalate stones [29]. These new findings may lead to new therapeutic targets for managing and preventing stones and would not have been possible without bringing investigators from different fields together.

Though saying little about the quality of the collaboration on outcomes such as academic culture and functioning or on training and mentoring, research collaborations are often measured through co-authorships of research papers. Indeed, the growth in collaborative science is reflected in author lists on scientific papers. Between 1981 and 2001, the average number of co-authors on a publication in the Proceedings of the National Academy of Sciences USA rose from 3.9 to 8.4 [30]. From 2013 to 2018, the number of papers in the Nature Index with more than a thousand authors surged from 0 to 100 [31]. Other metrics further illustrate the rise in the number of authors and of teams in publications (Fig. 9.1). Again, however, the number of authors on a publication does not necessarily imply a high level of cognitive unity or shared vision nor even a successful research collaboration. The increasing number of funding opportunity announcements requiring collaborative "interdisciplinary" or "transdisciplinary" research teams has caused concern about how this may encourage "fake collaborations," [32, 33] teams that may be put together in a "box-ticking" approach [32] without true collaborative processes. Concerns of this approach include an undermining of research integrity and transparency as well as the awarding of funds to less collaborative research teams at the expense of those that are more collaborative. Extremely short turn-around times for grant applications are cited as a major driver of this phenomenon.

Features of successful collaborations. The first ingredient in a successful collaboration is good collaborators. Individuals with shared goals and a cooperative spirit are good candidates. Ideal collaborators are individuals who (1) share characteristics of teams and groups, (2) recognize and value each other's unique expertise while maintaining a certain independence, (3) jointly agree upon common goals and implement them through mutual support, (4) build trust leading to open and honest dialogue, (5) recognize conflict is normal, and (6) jointly participate in decisions [36]. Second, a fully developed collaboration requires shared thinking and problem-solving such that participants are able to define the problem, understand

Fig. 9.1 Trends in number of authors (**A**) and percentage of international teams of authors on peer-reviewed scientific publications (**B**). Data for the figures were adapted from references [34, 35], respectively

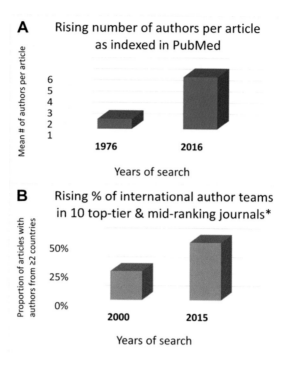

the expertise that each member brings to the team, agree on what the gaps in current knowledge are and on goals to address those gaps, and share responsibility to monitor progress in achieving the goals of the collaboration [37]. Third, accountability to each other, based on developing trust and interdependence (acknowledging that outcomes are contingent upon the actions of another) [38], thus forming the basis for cooperative behavior among individuals, are additional factors. Trust leads to cooperative behavior [39]. Communication and interaction are central to trust building [36]. Communication is most effective when collaborators work out in advance a "shared language," particularly when they are from different fields [26]. Fourth, the focus of the partnership revolves around shared objectives, not issues of power. When power structures are ignored, the possibility of having more open communication is increased, and the road is opened to build consensus on objectives [40]. Finally, leadership within collaborative research initiatives must be effective. Attributes that have been ascribed to effective leaders within research collaborations, especially in interdisciplinary and transdisciplinary research scenarios, include: respected stature as an investigator; empowerment-based leadership; ability to motivate others; "boundary-spanning;" encouraging; and good organizational skills [41, 42]. Other features of successful research collaborations are summarized (Fig. 9.2).

COLLABORATORS BEGIN WITH…

	- Mutual interests	- Collegiality
	- Deep trust	- Communication
	- Knowledge	- Flexibility

| Clinical example: | **A** | Clinical nutritionist | Urologist | Nephrologist |
| Academic example: | **B** | Clinician scientist | Basic scientist | Animal scientist |

AND INCORPORATE

ATTRIBUTES FAVORING SUCCESSFUL COLLABORATION
- Regular, frequent meetings
- Intellectual disagreement encouraged
- Credit and recognition shared
- Individuality is respected
- Expectations are adaptable

- Shared vision	- Shared planning
- Shared objective	- Shared thinking
- Shared passion	- Shared commitment

TO INTEGRATE

Expertise   Resources

TO DISCOVER

New knowledge
Improved processes

EXAMPLES OF RESEARCH OUTPUTS & OUTCOMES
- Models
- Prototypes
- Resources
- Products
- Assays
- Policies
- Procedures
- New hypotheses
- Abstracts
- Papers
- Manuscripts
- Research funding

TO CREATE

Research outputs and outcomes

ULTIMATELY LEADING TO

NEW KNOWLEDGE, ACADEMIC ACHIEVEMENT

Fig. 9.2 Model for academic collaboration (adapted from the model described and illustrated by Montiel-Overall in reference 21). As collaborators come together with trust, collegiality, and with shared academic or research interests, they develop shared objectives to be accomplished in the collaboration. As the work to be undertaken is planned and subdivided, each collaborator uses his/her unique expertise to complete his/her part. When all parts are combined, new knowledge and/or other outputs are created that could not otherwise have been created individually

Benefits and Challenges of Collaboration

Benefits of collaborations. Successful collaborations create new knowledge and insights. Collaborations have other benefits as well. Whether across laboratories in a single program or department or across different scientific or medical disciplines, data show higher productivity when basic and clinical research are done collaboratively [43]. Having connections to different groups increases heterogeneity of ideas and activities; and the breadth of these ties has been shown to predict innovation and creativity [44]. There may be implications of the size of collaborative research teams. By assessing large datasets from 1954 to 2014 from the Web of Science, the US Patent and Trademark Office, and GitHub—totaling hundreds of millions of articles, patents, and software products—Wu et al. concluded that the size of research teams mattered with respect to accomplishments. They found that larger teams were more productive and generated more translatable results than smaller teams. However, smaller teams were more likely to disrupt their fields with new concepts and ideas capable of challenging dogma and introducing new directions and opportunities [45]. Collaborative relationships can be a means of acquiring social capital and are therefore appropriate when that is the goal. Social capital is linked with academic success, including tenure [46], and career advancement. Social capital also directly aids the clinical process [47], improving patient care and satisfaction and also potentially enhancing the ability of clinical investigators to incorporate research into their work, in turn contributing to a learning healthcare system and generating data to drive evidence-based practice. In other cases, collaborations provide opportunities for collaborators that they would not otherwise have. For example, some senior faculty enjoy working with post-doctoral fellows and junior faculty to help them advance their careers or meet academic research goals. A desire to mentor students and faculty is a major motivation for some senior collaborators. Other benefits to individual collaborators include a feeling of contributing to something larger, the results of which potentially have greater significance compared to what each person could realize alone; opportunity to acquire new skills; and networking, which could lead to career advancement. Being able to work effectively with professionals from many different backgrounds can be a very marketable skill.

Challenges of collaborations. Although collaboration is increasingly encouraged in the academic setting, little formal training to develop these skills is available. As a result, many of us initiate collaborations without appropriate planning. Collaborations are not always easy to initiate or carry out. They can be cumbersome. At times it may feel that more work is created; indeed, more work usually is required. They may require uncomfortable discussions, such as about the productivity of individuals within the collaboration, funding, and authorship, and can lead to uncomfortable interactions. Putting together a collaboration with the most appropriate individuals may mean working with someone you don't know and/or whose methods are different than yours. Collaborators may have different work styles, which may contribute to questions or suspicions about commitment, work ethic, or output. The timescale for research may be longer than for a single-PI or unidisciplinary project as the more people that are involved, the more time must be spent on bringing people together to meet, exchange knowledge, make plans, and compile and interpret results. This process is often contraindicated by short turn-around times for grant applications. Identifying the best team leader(s) may be challenging. Strong collaborations usually require strong leadership with respect to organization, planning, communication, and conflict resolution. Individuals with these qualities may be lacking within certain collaborations. A challenge faced particularly by early-career stage investigators is potential lack of recognition for collaborative work. In its excellent policy report on collaborative academic research ("team science"), the United Kingdom's Academy of Medical Sciences found that "academic reward and recognition systems have failed to match the growth of team working," acknowledging the persistence of the long-held tradition of individual scholarship that prioritizes independence [48]. Indeed, the lack of recognition for one's contributions within a collaborative research team was cited as a major impediment to researchers considering participation, especially those in early career settings [48].

Potential Challenges in the practice of "Team Science" [34]

- Identifying the optimal group of investigators to address the questions of interest.
- Addressing issues of heterogeneity in combining data.
- Ensuring engagement, participation, and oversight of all collaborators.
- Agreeing on how to present and interpret results.
- Ensuring that all are appropriate recognized for their contributions.

Another problem relates to potential conflicts of interest that arise from collaboration. Definitions of "conflict of interest" vary between funders. Moreover, some definitions have changed over time. But one thing in common is that unbiased grant reviewers are sought to participate on scientific review panels. In order to ensure this, funding agencies frequently require that grant applicants disclose all co-authors and project collaborators. As research becomes more collaborative, these lists will grow. Investigators worry that collaboration will reduce the number of individuals who will be able to review their grant applications. This is a particular concern for those in areas of science that are small, nascent or emerging, or for which there are few experts. Fear exists even among investigators from different disciplines who may be considering inter- and transdisciplinary research teams, and this is related to grant review panels that are increasingly multi-disciplinary specifically because of the interdisciplinary research proposals to be reviewed. For these and other reasons, wariness of entering into collaborative relationships with other researchers may be an impediment for some investigators. Other challenges associated with research collaborations are summarized in the **sidebar**.

The Clinician Scientist Research Collaboration

The history of the physician-scientist is centuries old. Early observations by practitioners "in the field" led to multi-directional laboratory-based inquiries that generated foundational discoveries about human anatomy and physiology, organ function, biochemistry, and genetics. But the number of clinicians taking their discoveries into the lab to explore and address them—"from stethoscope to microscope"—has been in steady decline for a century or longer. Reasons for this include: a shift away from basic science in medical school training; extra time required to train as a scientist after medical school; lack of dedicated research experience and training in most medical residency programs; steep increases in the cost of medical training and personal debts that encourage early-career physicians to take more lucrative non-academic positions; increasing time demands of providing clinical care; financial burden on academic departments to support medical residency programs, resulting in demands on clinical staff to generate revenue; fewer academic physician-scientist mentors and role models; low rate of physician-scientist R01 renewals; and an overall decline in federal funding and institutional support for physicians' research [49–52]. Although professional medical organizations, such as the American Urological Association, and multiple federal funding agencies have created initiatives to promote physician-scientists, physicians engaged in scientific research account for a mere 1.5% of the physician workforce [52]. Thus, the efforts of these organizations may be insufficient in reversing the trend.

These barriers should not preclude physicians' engagement in research, however. Because basic scientists are now expected to be more involved in clinical/translational research, clinical partners are needed. Demands on basic research scientists to produce translatable research results are higher than ever. Thus translational research may be an ideal forum for building interdisciplinary and transdisciplinary research teams. Yet many, if not most basic scientists, have little to no access to human subjects nor experience in conducting human subjects research (e.g., to acquire and use biological samples, to collect samples with clinical information attached). Some have insufficient appreciation for the clinical relevance of their work. Others perceive their research, which is often highly controlled, as more rigorous than the goal-directed or descriptive research often conducted in clinical settings [53]. In a survey of nearly 900 basic scientists from four major metropolitan areas in the USA and Europe, Sorrentino et al. found a negative correlation between involvement in basic research and motivation for the "health benefit to society." Furthermore, they found a positive correlation between PIs' involvement in basic research and their rejection of the requirement to discuss the health benefit potential in research proposals [54]. This suggests lower interest in engaging in translational research and/or indifference to or lack of interest in the future health-related impact of their research. Indeed, survey results of the same study demonstrated that nearly 50% of respondents agreed with the statement about grant applications that "writing the sections discussing potential future health benefits takes too much time" [54].

These twin problems—constraints on physicians and other clinicians from engaging in scientific research and on basic research scientists to engage in translational science—represent two sides of the same coin. Collaborative research teams that fully recognize the attributions, strengths, and contributions of both sectors and that offer tangible benefits to both are needed. Hobin and Galbraith point out that it is in the interest of both sides to engage in translational science:

> (T)he clinical potential of bench discoveries is more likely to be realized when basic scientists have opportunities to interact and collaborate with their clinical research and clinician colleagues, support from their institutions to pursue translational leads, and training, guidance, and resources throughout the process [55].

My Experiences with Collaboration

My graduate school training, initiated after earning becoming a registered dietitian nutritionist (RDN), was conventional in the sense that the goal was to become an independent investigator. My research was a combination of basic and applied science and involved the use of animal models in retinoid assessment methodology. Near the end of the Ph.D. process, I considered a post-doc within the field. But by that time I had accumulated nearly 6 years of experience as a RDN from serving as the clinical nutrition member of the half-day, weekly, multidisciplinary stone prevention team at the University Hospital. During those years, I experienced first-hand the rise in the stone clinic's visibility within the region. Patient referrals were increasing, and a new endourology fellowship with dual emphases in clinical management and research in metabolic stone disease was on its fourth fellow. Though created by a urologist and housed in a urology clinic, the stone clinic was staffed by two senior nephrologists (Dr. Richard Rieselbach and Dr. Thomas Steele) with a special interest in kidney stones. Their knowledge and willingness to pass it along formed an early foundation in my understanding of stone disease.

Against this backdrop, thanks to a cadre of clinician and basic scientists who contributed to a rapidly increasing body of literature beginning in the 1980s and continuing through the 2000s, much was learned about the role of diet and stones. Indeed, using the search terms "diet" and urolithiasis," the number of PubMed-indexed publications related to the role of nutritional factors in kidney stones from 1946 to 2018 increased from a mean of 4/year to nearly 70/year (Fig. 9.3). It was within this context that clinical nutrition therapy as part of the medical management of stones was considered a critical and indispensable attribute of our stone clinic and, as such, required the specialized skills of a dedicated RDN (clinical nutrition FTE from the hospital's clinical nutrition service was provided from the inception of the UW Health Metabolic Stone Clinic in 1995). It was also within this context that a role for clinical nutrition research in stone prevention

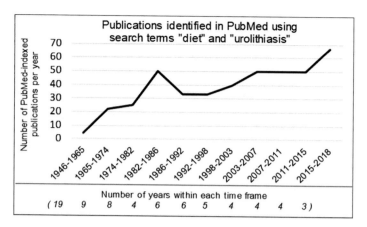

Fig. 9.3 Rise in number of PubMed-indexed publications related to "diet" and "urolithiasis." Data show mean number of publications per year (y-axis) within time frames shown on x-axis. Search results were not filtered in any way; some publications are reports of clinical studies while others are mechanistic, some of which were animal or in vitro studies. Note that the time frames are not equally distributed

became more visible. By the time I completed my Ph.D. and was offered a scientist position within urology, I saw the translatable potential of the study of nutrition and its effects on stone formation and growth and realized that I wanted to be part of contributing to that science.

Developing a collaborative mindset. From the beginning of my academic career, I was fortunate that Dr. Stephen Y. Nakada, then urology division chief and now department chair, fostered a collaborative working association instead of the more traditional "employer-employee" relationship. Because of my knowledge and training in nutrition, and because I had demonstrated for several years a passion for the nutritional management of patients with stones, he invited me to contribute as much as I wanted toward the development of a clinical stone research program within the department. Being valued for what I could "bring to the table" played a foundational role in developing the collaborative mindset I would need in finding a place for myself in urology and ways to make meaningful contributions. Perhaps equally as critical was the willingness among my urology colleagues to accept my contributions and ideas as important. The research program we developed has provided significant research opportunities and unique experiences to numerous endourology fellows, a number of interesting research findings, and advances in the way patients in our stone clinic are managed.

My collaborative experiences. I have enjoyed collaborative relationships with several individuals over time and have learned many lessons. In my early years as a scientist, I continued a collaboration I cultivated while in graduate school. By participating in various journal clubs and discussion groups, I maintained contact with a swine expert on campus, with whom I had collaborated on several studies related to my Ph.D. When I obtained funding for a swine study in my new area of research, I had a ready-made collaboration that greatly expedited my progress. Not only were my needs met, but my collaborator's need to train his students was also met as he introduced them to my work and as I was able to incorporate some of them into my studies. One of the students who helped me with sample collection and preparation eventually became a Ph.D-prepared veterinarian whom I am now mentoring in her K12 scholar project. A lesson I learned from this experience was the power of regular interactions, such as journal clubs, and to keep relationships and collaborations going through times of no active research. I also learned that collaborations benefit when participating parties each have something to gain above and beyond the products of the research itself.

Through my work in the Department of Urology with Stephen Nakada, I learned other lessons about collaborating. One is the importance of regular, ongoing meetings to track and review progress on agreed-upon tasks, goals, and objectives. Even when it seems there is nothing new to discuss, that regular meeting serves as an aid to staying sharp and developing new ideas. In working collaboratively with both inexperienced and experienced investigators, I learned that people stay motivated when they get something out of it, whatever that means for them. It could be authorship on a paper, an abstract and being able to present it at a meeting, or something else, such as training or the opportunity to mentor. As I work with students, I apply this lesson by thinking about what drives them and then try to use that to maintain their motivation. The freedom to disagree and to encourage intellectual debate is another important aspect to successfully working together. I am fortunate that this is a characteristic of several of my academic relationships. It is not uncommon in our endourology research group meetings, for example, to begin with opposing ideas and then work through them. Sometimes we end up somewhere in the middle, and other times one or more of us have the flexibility and open-mindedness to change positions. In other cases, such as in many journal club meetings with various colleagues, intellectual debates and differences were made fun. This helped to create a culture of learning and curiosity and made the students who were part of those discussions open up and more likely to participate. Finally, allowing people to work in the fashion that works for them has emerged in my experience as a feature of a good collaboration. This means being adaptable and willing to adjust expectations. Meeting preferences differ (time, location, frequency) as do communication styles (longer vs. shorter meetings, Zoom vs. telephone contact, etc.), and it helps when collaborating parties identify what's most important to them as well as the things they are less concerned with. This abets the process of compromise, which is inevitably necessary in most teams.

Academic Research Collaborations in the COVID Era

Over the past 2 years, collaborative research initiatives—even those within a single institution—were affected by physical isolation mandates put in place to slow the transmission of the COVID-19 virus. Investigators already engaged in multi-institutional research collaborations, including multinational, were somewhat better prepared as many had already been utilizing technology to communicate and cooperate. Most, however, had to quickly learn new ways to have progress meetings, engage in discussion, and share knowledge. Even before COVID, challenges for virtual teams were documented [56]. While largely related to geographically distributed corporate work places, many of these challenges became familiar to those in the academic world. Issues arose related to, for example, reduced motivation of team members due to social isolation, slower or halted research progress, difficulties in establishing and maintaining trust, and the loss of unintentional but critical information exchanges from face-to-face contact [55]. While some of the problems encountered in virtual meetings are new, others are problems that beset research networking and collaboration even in the best of times. De Lora and Termini developed a "virtual toolbox" for maintaining research collaborations [57], which may provide useful ideas and strategies for virtual collaboration.

Within the collaborative benign genitourinary research consortium I lead through a U24 "interactions core" mechanism (U24-DK-127726), we recognized in leadership meetings at the start of the pandemic that opportunities for consortium-affiliated K12 Scholars and other trainees to be invited to speak at meetings and conferences would be limited. These are often important networking, resume-building, and collaboration-forming opportunities for early-stage investigators seeking academic positions. Within the consortium (known as CAIRIBU—Collaborating for the Advancement of Interdisciplinary Research in Benign Urology), we developed a response to this problem by creating a mechanism for monthly virtual seminars. These have been successful and well-attended and even garnered attendance of individuals from broader geographic and disciplinary ranges than would have been possible in a face-to-face format.

In addition to enhancing the training and visibility of early-career stage investigators in benign urology, an important goal of CAIRIBU is to foster and encourage the formation of interdisciplinary research interest groups. In pre-pandemic times, we may have organized an in-person event to which we would have invited key players and others interested in a certain area of research. It may have been deemed successful but likely would have included only those available to set aside several days of travel and, thus, excluded a few experts whose schedules tend to be less flexible. Because of the pandemic and our newly-founded expertise in virtual meetings, we organized a kick-off event for a particular area of benign urology research in which we are interested and have sustained subsequent virtual discussions that include a wide geographic and disciplinary breadth and a solid mix of trainees and experts. The number of participants has actually grown over time. The hope is that this momentum can foment the formation of small collaborative "collectives" that will create proposals for novel and fundable research projects. In small breakout rooms, we envision that investigator groups will work on various stages of their proposals and then re-convene in the "larger" virtual room to get immediate feedback from others. Several iterations of this process may result in the kind of highly-meritorious research proposals that are needed in benign urology research. We know that a key aspect of collaborative science is trust and that this need is most pronounced during the initial stage of the collaboration [57]. Much has been written about the inability of virtual meetings to convey the kinds of body language, facial expression, and voice inflection cues that help people build trust [58]. While not a perfect surrogate for face-to-face interactions, we responded to this potential challenge in our new research interest group by prioritizing getting to know each other. We have accomplished this by taking time at the beginning of each meeting to hear from five to six investigators, hoping eventually to hear from everyone involved. In addition, we are collecting and archiving these "bios" for posting on our website. It is possible that we may conclude in this case that the virtual collaboration format was actually superior with respect to attracting and maintaining the involvement of a variety of investigators and in achieving our goals.

Summary

Collaborative science is a means to producing knowledge that would otherwise never happen [9], especially now when research questions are larger and more involved and when both clinicians and scientists are ever-more specialized. This stands in contrast to the traditional paradigm of independent investigator. When multifaceted expertise is required, groups of researchers who join with a common vision to solve problems bring their individual knowledge and expertise. Career advancement systems and other forms of recognition will hopefully acknowledge and include the accomplishments derived from successful research collaborations. Funding announcements for collaborative awards, especially those involving complex teams of interdisciplinary personnel, will hopefully lengthen the turn-around times for grant applications and/or support investigators who are taking the preliminary steps of forming substantive and meaningful collaborations. Key features of successful collaborations and some of the lessons learned are summarized (Table 9.2).

Table 9.2 Key features of successful collaborations and lessons learned. This list, which appears in no particular order, draws upon the cited literature and on personal experiences

Features/lessons	Rationale
Recognize and value each other's unique expertise while maintaining a certain independence	Creates a culture of respect and individuality, the latter of which promotes interdependence (acknowledging that outcomes are contingent upon the actions of another)
Recognize conflict is normal	Anticipating this may prompt preemptive discussions and decision-making, which are usually better had when things are going well
Jointly participate in decisions	Avoids unnecessary conflict; promotes investment by all participants and a cooperative spirit
Intellectual differences and debate are encouraged	Promotes a culture of learning; creates a safe space for participation, and builds trust
Allow people to work in the ways that are the most productive for them	Maximizes collaborative outcomes when everyone participating at high level; individuals feel respected
Be flexible and willing to adjust expectations	There might not be only one way for something to be done
Have regularly scheduled, ongoing meetings	Promotes accountability to one another, interdependence, and mutual responsibility
Realize that each individual needs something out of the collaboration	Examples include shared credit, authorship, education, opportunity to mentor, academic recognition, funding, access to resources, labor, social capital
Avoid unnecessary power structures and/or suspend power relations during active collaboration	Promotes open and honest communication; encourages a feeling of shared empowerment, enhancing individuals' motivation and participation

References

1. Wuchty S, Jones BF, Uzzi B. The increasing dominance of teams in production of knowledge. Science. 2007;316:1036–9.
2. Tachibana C. Navigating collaborative grant research. Science careers. https://doi.org/10.1126/science.opms.rl300136. Retrieved from: https://www.sciencemag.org/sites/default/files/documents/printed-publications/13%20Sept%20Faculty%20Feature_0.pdf (2013). Accessed 30 Dec 2018.
3. Committee on the Science of Team Science; Board on Behavioral, Cognitive, and Sensory Sciences; Division of Behavioral and Social Sciences and Education; National Research Council; Cooke NJ, Hilton ML, editors. Enhancing the Effectiveness of Team Science. Washington (DC): National Academies Press (US). 15 July 2015. 9, Funding and Evaluation of Team Science. Retrieved from: https://www.ncbi.nlm.nih.gov/books/NBK310379/. Accessed 30 Dec 2018.
4. Petterson MB, Longhurst C, Yu J-PJ. Measuring interdisciplinarity of biomedical research, medical specialty performance, and implications for radiology: a retrospective review of 2.6 million citations. Clin Imaging. 2021;80:322–328.

5. National Institute of Diabetes and Digestive and Kidney Diseases. Executive summary, NIDDK extramural funding trends and support of guiding principles. Retrieved from: https://www.niddk.nih.gov/research-funding/funded-grants-grant-history/funding-trends-support-core-values. Accessed 12 Jan 2021.
6. Conte ML, Liu J, Schnell S, Omary MB. Globalization and changing trends of biomedical research output. JCI Insight. 2017;2: e95206.
7. Cline H, Coolen L, de Vries S, Hyman S, Segal R, Steward O. Recognizing team science contributions in academic hiring, promotion, and tenure. J Neurosci. 2020;40:6662–3.
8. McHale S, Damayanthi R, DiazGranados D, Bagshaw D, Schienke E, Blank AE. Promotion and tenure policies for team science at colleges/schools of medicine. J Clin Transl Sci. 2019;3:245–52.
9. Denbo S. Whose work is it really? Collaboration and the question of credit. Perspectives on history. Retrieved from: https://www.historians.org/publications-and-directories/perspectives-on-history/february-2017/whose-work-is-it-really-collaboration-and-the-question-of-credit (2017). Accessed 29 Dec 2018.
10. Schöttle A, Haghsheno S, Gehbauer: defining cooperation and collaboration in the context of lean construction. Proceedings IGLC-22; June 2014:1269–80.
11. Bozeman B, Fay D, Slade CP. Research collaboration in universities and academic entrepreneurship: the state-of-the-art. J Technol Transf. 2013;38:1–67.
12. Baldwin RG, Chang DA. Collaborating to learn, learning to collaborate. Peer Rev. 2007;9:26–30.
13. Bronstein LR. A model for interdisciplinary collaboration. Soc Work. 2003;48:297–306.
14. Dillenbourg P. What do you mean by 'collaborative learning?' In: Dillenbourg P, editor. Collaborative-learning: cognitive and computational approaches. Oxford, UK: Elsevier Publishing; 1999. p. 1–19.
15. Hardin SR. Michael Schrage and collaboration. Bull Am Soc Inf Sci. 1998; 6–8.
16. Macrina FL, Dynamic issues in scientific integrity,. collaborative research. Washington, DC: American Academy of Microbiology; 1995.
17. Roschelle J, Teasley SD. The construction of shared knowledge in collaborative problem solving. In: O'Malley C, editor. Computer supported collaborative learning. Berlin, Heidelberg: Springer; 1995. p. 69–96.
18. Mattessich PW, Monsey BR. Collaboration: what makes it work? St. Paul, MN: Amherst H. Wilder Foundation;1992.
19. Wood DJ, Gray B. Toward a comprehensive theory of collaboration. J Appl Behav Sci. 1991;27:139–62.
20. Appley DG, Winder AE. An evolving definition of collaboration and some implications for the world of work. J Appl Behav Sci. 1977;13:279–91.
21. Meadows AJ. Scientific collaboration and status. In: Communication in science. Butterworths: London; 1974. p. 172–206.
22. Stember M. Advancing the social sciences through the interdisciplinary enterprise. Soc Sci J. 1991;28:1–14.
23. Miller EC, Leffert L. Building cross-disciplinary research collaborations. Stroke. 2019;49: e43–5.
24. Campbell D. Reforms as experiment Am Psychol. 1969;24(409):429.
25. Stein Z. Modeling the demands of interdisciplinarity: toward a framework for evaluating interdisciplinary endeavors. Integral Review. 2007;4:92–107.
26. Bennett LM, Gadlin H. Collaboration and team science: from theory to practice. J Investig Med. 2012;60:768–75.
27. Jones BF, Wuchty S, Uzzi B. Multi-university research teams: shifting impact, geography, and stratification in science. Science. 2008;322:1259–62.
28. Bennett LM, Gadlin H, Levine-Finley S. Collaboration and team science: a field guide. National Institutes of Health. Bethesda, MD. Retrieved from https://www.hopkinsmedicine.org/women_science_medicine/_pdfs/team%20science%20field%20guide.pdf   (2010). Accessed 31 Dec 2018.

29. Sivaguru M, Saw JL, Williams JC Jr, Lieske JC, Krambeck AE, Romero MF, Chia N, Schwaderer AL, Alcalde RE, Bruce WJ, Wildman DE, Fried GA, Werth CJ, Reeder RJ, Yau PM, Sanford RA, Fouke BW. Geobiology reveals how human kidney stones dissolve *in vivo*. Sci Rep. 2018;8:13731.
30. Börner K, Maru JT, Goldstone RL. The simultaneous evolution of author and paper networks. PNAS. 2004;101:5266–73.
31. Mallapaty S. Paper authorship goes hyper. Nature Index News. Retrieved from: https://www.natureindex.com/news-blog/paper-authorship-goes-hyper/ (2018). Accessed 29 Nov 2021.
32. Hessels RS, Kingstone A. Fake collaborations: interdisciplinary science can undermine research integrity. PsyArXiv. Retrieved from: https://doi.org/10.31234/osf.io/rqwea (2019). Accessed 29 Nov 2021.
33. Conroy G. The push for interdisciplinary teams can lead to fake collaborations. Nature Index News. Retrieved from https://www.natureindex.com/news-blog/push-interdisciplinary-teams-science-research-can-lead-fake-collaborations (2020). Accessed 04 Dec 2021.
34. Fontanarosa P, Bauchner H, Flanagin A. Authorship and team science. JAMA. 2017;318:2433–7.
35. U.S. National Library of Medicine: Number of authors per MEDLINE/PubMed citation. Retrieved from http://www.nlm.nih.gov/bsd/authors1.html (2017). Accessed 29 Dec 2018.
36. Montiel-Overall P. Toward a theory of collaboration for teachers and librarians. School Library Media Research 2005;8. ISSN 1523–4320. Retrieved from: http://www.ala.org/aasl/sites/ala.org.aasl/files/content/aaslpubsandjournals/slr/vol8/SLMR_TheoryofCollaboration_V8.pdf. Accessed 30 Dec 2018.
37. Graesser A, Kuo B-C, Liao C-H. Complex problem solving in assessments of collaborative problem solving. J Intell. 2017;5:10.
38. Sheppard BH, Sherman DM. The grammars of trust: a model and general implications. Acad Manag Rev. 1998;23:422–37.
39. Jones GR, George JM. The experience and evolution of trust: implications for cooperation and teamwork. Acad Manag Rev. 1998;23:531–46.
40. Lee SS, Jabloner A. Institutional culture is the key to team science. Nat Biotechnol. 2017;35:1212–4.
41. Calhoun WJ, Wooten K, Bhavnani S, Anderson KE, Freeman J, Brasier AR. The CTSA as an exemplar framework for developing multidisciplinary translational teams. Clin Transl Sci. 2013;6:60–71.
42. Elkins T, Keller RT. Leadership in research and development organizations: a literature review and conceptual framework. Leadersh Q. 2003;14:587–606.
43. Antonio-García MT, López-Navarro I, Rey-Rocha J. Determinants of success for biomedical researchers: a perception-based study in a health science research environment. Scientometrics. 2014;101:1747–79.
44. Shalley CE, Gilson LL. What leaders need to know: a review of social and contextual factors than can foster or hinder creativity. Leadersh Q. 2004;15:33–53.
45. Wu L, Wang D, Evans JA. Large teams develop and small teams disrupt science and technology. Nature. 2019;566:378–82.
46. Lutter M, Schröder M. Who becomes a tenured professor, and why? Panel data evidence from German sociology, 1980–2013. MPIfG Discussion Paper. 2014;14:1–25.
47. Perzynski AT, Caron A, Margolius D, Sudano JJ Jr. Primary care practice workplace social capital: a potential secret sauce for improved staff well-being and patient experience J Patient Exp. 2018. https://doi.org/10.1177/2374373518777742.
48. Academy of Medical Sciences: Improving recognition of team science contributions in biomedical research careers. London, UK. Retrieved from: https://acmedsci.ac.uk/viewFile/56defebabba91.pdf (2016). Accessed 19 Jan 2019.
49. Eberli D, Atala A. Basic science research in urology training. Indian J Urol. 2009;25:217–20.
50. Permar SR, Ward RA, Barrett KJ, Freel SA, Gbadegesin RA, Kontos CD, Hu PJ, Hartmann KE, Williams CS, Vyas JM. Addressing the physician-scientist pipeline: strategies to integrate research into clinical training programs. J Clin Invest. 2020;130:1058–61.

51. Liu EA, Wang SY, Rao RC. Sustaining independent careers in vision research: demographics and success in second R01 attainment among clinician-scientists from 1985 to 2019. Trans Vis Sci Tech. 2020;9:32.

52. Jain MK, Cheung VG, Utz PJ, Kobilka BK, Yamada T, Lefkowitz R. Saving the endangered physician-scientist – a plan for accelerating medical breakthroughs. N Engl J Med. 2019;381:399–402.

53. Hobin JA, Deschamps AM, Bockman R, Cohen S, Dechow P, Eng C, Galey W, Morris M, Prabhakar S, Raj U, Rubenstein P, Smith JA, Stover P, Sung N, Talman W, Galbraith R. Engaging basic scientists in translational research: identifying opportunities, overcoming obstacles. J Transl Med. 2012;10:72.

54. Sorrentino C, Boggio A, Confalonieri S, Hemenway D, Scita G, Ballabeni A. Increasing both the public health potential of basic research and the scientist satisfaction: an international survey of bio-scientists. F1000Research 2016;5:56.

55. Hobin JA, Galbraith RA. Engaging basic scientists in translational research. FASEB J. 2012;26:2227–30.

56. Morrison-Smith S, Ruiz J. Challenges and barriers in virtual teams: a literature review. SN Applied Sciences. 2020;2:1096.

57. De Lora JA, Termini CM. Synthesis and assembly of virtual collaborations. Trends Biochem Sci. 2020;45:823–5.

58. Bos N, Olson J, Gergle D, Olson G, Wright Z. Effects of four computer-mediated communications channels on trust development. In: Terveen L, Wixon D, Comstock E, Sasse A, editors. Proceedings of the conference on human factors in computing systems, vol. 4, 1st ed. 2002. p. 135–14.

Chapter 10
Patient Satisfaction

Sarah E. Tevis and Nizar N. Jarjour

Background

Satisfaction is the fulfillment of one's wishes, expectations, or needs, or the pleasure derived from this. It can be viewed as a measure of how happy a person is with a given situation, which is often difficult to gauge during daily interactions with people. This is even more difficult to decipher as a surgeon interacting with a patient, perhaps one you are meeting for the first time. Many of us have been surprised to hear that a patient complained about their care after we interacted with them seemingly without incident. Therefore, a number of standardized tools have been developed to examine how satisfied patients are with their care. The data obtained can be harnessed to change our practice and shore up deficiencies to improve patient care and satisfaction.

Patient satisfaction is a quantitative measure of how patient experience, as they progress through the care process, compares with their expectations. This differs from other commonly used metrics. **Patient-reported outcome measures** (PROMs) are any report of the status of a patients' health condition or health behavior that comes directly from a patient without interpretation by a clinician. This includes tools that measure health-related quality of life and symptoms. **Patient-centered care** is described as safe, effective, timely, efficient, and equitable care. **Patient experience** encompasses the cumulative evaluation of the patient with the health care system and providers; with particular focus on relationships, trust, and peace of mind.

S. E. Tevis
Department of Surgery, University of Colorado, Aurora, CO, USA

N. N. Jarjour (✉)
Department of Medicine, University of Wisconsin School of Medicine and Public Health, Madison, WI, USA
e-mail: nnj@medicine.wisc.edu

History of Patient Satisfaction

In 1999, the Institute of Medicine published "To Err is Human: Building a Safer Health System", which described thousands of deaths due to medical errors in the United States [1]. While the healthcare quality improvement organized efforts started years earlier, the safety of medical care was not publicly scrutinized until the publication of this report. Health care organizations, insurers, government agencies, and accrediting bodies responded with interventions to improve safety and quality of care in the United States, which included a focus on involving patients in their care. In 2002, the Centers for Medicare and Medicaid Services (CMS) and the Agency for Healthcare Research and Quality (AHRQ) joined forces to develop the Hospital Consumer Assessment of Healthcare Providers and Systems (HCAHPS) patient satisfaction survey [2]. HCAHPS measures patients' perceptions of their hospital experience via a survey instrument and data collection methodology, the results of which allow consumers to objectively compare hospitals. The increased transparency through public reporting of survey results motivates hospitals to address patients' concerns and improve quality of care. The psychometric properties of the survey were validated, and the HCAHPS survey was endorsed by the National Quality Forum (NQF) in 2005.

Hospitals have placed added focus on improving HCAHPS scores as patient satisfaction is now tied to Medicare reimbursement. The Affordable Care Act of 2010 established the Hospital Value Based Purchasing program. HCAHPS scores fulfill the Patient and Caregiver Experience of Care/Care Coordination domain that comprises 25% of the Total Performance Score in the CMS Hospital Value Based Purchasing program. Importantly, patient feedback can lead to improvements in care delivery and better outcomes. Patients who are satisfied with their care will return themselves and recommend the hospital or physician to friends and family. Patients can now reach a large number of people very quickly using social media and online platforms and, as a result, they are increasingly being considered as customers.

Measurement Tools

The HCAHPS survey, like other standardized patient satisfaction questionnaires, aims to quantify subjective opinion based on evaluation at multiple patient touchpoints [3]. The survey consists of 29 items administered to a random sample of adult patients discharged from medical, surgical, or obstetric services. The survey includes global questions about overall rating of the hospital on a scale of 0–10 and willingness to recommend the hospital from definitely yes to definitely no. The remainder of the questions, each with multiple choice answers, asks about interactions and communications with physicians and nurses, ease of access such as appointment scheduling, responsiveness of hospital staff, pain management, and communication about medicines, discharge instructions, and environmental factors such as cleanliness of the facility. Each question like "During this hospital stay, how often did doctors listen carefully to you" has these possible responses: never, sometimes, usually, and always. "Top box" scores indicate the percentage of patients who chose the most favorable answer for each question. For the "doctors listen carefully to you" question above, the "top box" score would be the percentage of patients who responded "always". Other questions inquired about frequency of doctors "explaining things in a way you could understand", and "treat you with courtesy and respect". The results of the survey are adjusted based on patient case mix and are reported quarterly by CMS. The Hospital Compare website (www. medicare.gov/hospitalcompare)   administered   by   CMS   publically   reports hospital-specific scores and compares scores across hospitals [4].

Patient voices can be captured by other mechanisms including patient councils and representatives, consumer apps, social media, and online reviews or patient communities. Popular social media and online outlets include: Facebook, LinkedIn, YouTube, Twitter, Instagram, Angi, Yelp!, SnapChat, as well as various blogs and websites. Hospitals and physicians are using social media more commonly to increase brand awareness and loyalty and to educate patients and the community. A consistent social media presence with valuable information and reputable followers reinforces to patients that their provider is an expert in the field and helps providers build a positive reputation. Many patients use the internet and social media to find hospitals and providers. Researchers have examined patient postings on social media groups to evaluate patient satisfaction with specific procedures. The use of online tools has the potential to improve communication between patients and their doctors and improve access to, and satisfaction with, care. While teenagers and 20-year olds have historically made up the majority of social media communities, today your 80-year-old bladder cancer patient is likely engaging on social media, which can be an important venue to share information, engage patients, and perhaps improve patient satisfaction.

What Correlates With High Satisfaction?

As patient satisfaction is studied more, we are learning about how institutional, process measures, and provider characteristics influence satisfaction scores [2]. Figure 10.1 summarizes many factors that have been found to be associated with high patient satisfaction. An institutional culture of safety encourages reporting patient safety events and focuses on providing safe, quality care by high-performing teams. Patient satisfaction has been shown to correlate with a focus on safety, staffing, team work, organizational learning, timely communication of errors, and non-punitive response to error.

Provider characteristics, interpersonal skills, and care team collaboration that are evident to the patient and family can all influence patient satisfaction. Patient satisfaction is enhanced when patients and their families feel that all health team

Fig. 10.1 Predictors of patient satisfaction

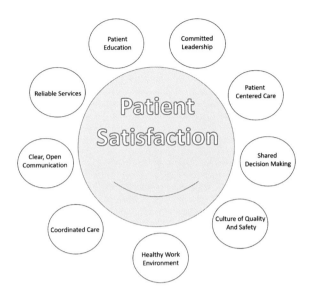

members treat them with dignity and respect, make them a priority, and listen to their concerns. Both physician and nursing burnout have been found to be inversely associated with satisfaction scores, highlighting the need to care for our staff in order to optimize patient care. When patients and families feel there is a caring team of physicians and staff who are communicating and working well together to provide patient-centered care, they are more likely to be satisfied.

Process and quality measures have been studied in relation to patient satisfaction, specifically the Hospital Quality Alliance (HQA) measures and the Healthcare Effectiveness Data and Information Set (HEDIS). HQA measures evaluate compliance with best practices for acute myocardial infarction, heart failure, and pneumonia. HEDIS measures monitor primary and secondary prevention and behavioral health care. Multiple studies have identified a positive correlation between HQA disease-specific process measures and patient satisfaction scores on the HCAHPS survey. A study of the HEDIS measures found higher patient satisfaction in numerous domains correlated with HEDIS process measure compliance.

While HCAHPS survey results have been extensively studied, less is known about predictors of satisfaction in the surgical patient population. An evaluation of >370,000 patients undergoing a major extirpative cancer surgery [9] found modest, but statistically significant correlations between high satisfaction on the HCAHPS survey and low complication rates ($p < 0.001$), readmissions ($p < 0.001$), and mortality ($p < 0.001$). A study of adult surgical patients requiring an overnight admission at a single academic institution [10] found that 72% of patients provided "top box" scores for overall physician satisfaction based on the Consumer Assessment of Healthcare Providers and Systems Surgical Care (S-CAHPS) survey, which focuses on patient satisfaction with surgeons, anesthesiologists, surgical staff, and surgical care. Independent predictors of "top box" responses on the S-CAHPS survey included preoperative communication (OR 6.8, 95% CI 2.9–16.1) and day of surgery attentiveness (OR 5.4, 95% CI 2.2–13.4). A study of >46,000 surgical patients with genitourinary cancer [11] did not find an association between high satisfaction on the HCAHPS survey and death, disposition status, medical complications, or surgical complications. The authors did note that patients' satisfaction was decreased with prolonged hospital stay (OR 0.77, 95% CI 0.64–0.92) and nursing sensitive complications (OR 0.85, 95% CI 0.72–0.99), which included venous thromboembolism, mobility related events, and sepsis. More work is needed to better delineate what influences patient satisfaction for patients undergoing surgery.

How to Improve Satisfaction Scores

The white paper by the Institute for Healthcare Improvement (IHI) on Achieving an Exceptional Patient and Family Experience of Inpatient Hospital Care is an excellent resource for administrators, physicians, and staff seeking to learn more about how to improve patient satisfaction [12]. Providers should be open to receiving patient satisfaction information in a variety of forms and should not write off certain sources, as any information about what patients think is helpful. This may include HCAHPS data, other standardized surveys, online patient reviews, patient-reported outcomes, or patient comments on social media.

Patients put their trust in their surgeons at an incredibly vulnerable time and, therefore, they are looking for compassionate care that addresses their physical and emotional needs. Patients present with a wide variation in health care literacy, however, even the most educated patients may have trouble processing and synthesizing information during a stressful time. Flexible teaching techniques and tools (visual aids, analogies, handouts, videos, web links) should be utilized to adapt to how individual patients learn best. Physicians come to the clinic visit with an "agenda"—we want to obtain information, examine the patient, and present our surgical plan. While patients may have a different expectations, physicians need to **listen** to patient (and family) concerns to fully engage in a clinical care relationship based on shared understanding and decision making. When physicians are not attentive or are constantly interrupting a patient, the patient does not feel listened to. Consequently, trust is not built and the critical personal connection with the patient cannot be established creating an obstacle to optimal care. Conversely, when patients and families are treated with respect and empathy, they will trust the healthcare team and be more engaged in their own care. Patients and families can be engaged in their own care with shared decision-making, being encouraged to ask questions and participate as much as they would like in their own care, thereby collaborating to develop common goals and treatment plans. Improving satisfaction isn't about being nice or giving patients everything they want, it is about taking the time to listen, communicate, and partner with patients and families for the best outcomes. Therefore, avoiding topics such as weight loss or smoking cessation or prescribing unnecessary medications such as antibiotics or pain medications, in an effort to please patient is not only ill advised, it is unethical. Physicians have a duty to discuss sensitive matters respectfully with their patients using clear language and teaching aids to ensure understanding. For example, if weight loss is important to reduce surgical complications, take time to explain that. Physicians can specifically explain why a lifestyle modification is important for the patient's surgical care. For example, excessive abdominal weight pushes on the diaphragm leaving less room for the lung to expand and leading to greater risk of post-operative atelectasis and pneumonia. Be realistic when giving specific expectations to patients and be encouraging of their effort while avoiding the tendency to show disappointment when they are unable to reach goals such as weight loss or smoking cessation.

Communication is especially important for surgical patients who need to adequately understand the risks and benefits of a surgical procedure as part of the informed consent process and to have appropriate expectations of the potential outcomes. Some specific examples where communication and shared decision-making is key in urologic surgery include setting expectations for patients with incontinence secondary to pelvic floor weakness, deciding when to obtain and how to act on PSA results, and discussing the risk associated with specific procedures such as risk of incontinence and erectile dysfunction after prostatectomy. Medical errors should be immediately disclosed and apologized for, because patients deserve honesty from the surgeon in whom they placed their trust. In addition to having clear, open communication with patients, physicians need to communicate well with the entire health care team. Patients may tell a medical student, resident, MA, or RN things they don't want to "bother" their surgeon with. If you have a good relationship with your clinical team and make it clear that you want to hear their thoughts, you may learn information from your team that patients are hesitant to share with you. Patients can tell when care is well coordinated, thus it is important to do your part to ensure there is clear communication within and between teams and reviewing conversations with consultants or what a night nurse had written in his or her report with patients. Patients and families cannot tell if your anastomosis was sewn perfectly, but they can tell if your communication with the cardiology consultant is poor or if nursing staff does not know the plan for the day. When HCFA began reporting hospital mortality data more than two decades ago hospitals with clearly higher mortalities saw no significant decrease in their patient volumes, suggesting that patients, in general, make their decisions based on personal values of the service they receive not the objective technical quality of care. It is very important to establish a connection when examining a patient by making eye contact, calling them by name, expressing kindness with words and gestures, and considering the whole person not just their illness. Attention to their privacy, dignity and responding appropriately to their concerns are crucial to ensuring a good patient experience.

Good communication with the care team can also improve employee satisfaction and thereby improve patient satisfaction. Having satisfied nurses improves patient satisfaction scores. Creating a healthy work environment for staff enables the recruitment and retention of staff with values that will ensure patient-centered, high-quality care. As a physician, you can influence working conditions and create joy in the workplace by making sure staff have the resources and skill they need to provide quality care, acknowledging good work and successes, and rewarding staff who go above and beyond for patients.

Patients want to know they will receive high quality, reliable care. This includes the ability to schedule appointments in a timely manner, staff that are available and responsive, and limited wait times for appointments, getting questions answered, and obtaining results. The hospital environment should also support healing with accessible parking or valet services and quiet comfortable patient waiting and care areas. A supportive environment decreases stress and improves the overall patient experience, which leads to greater patient satisfaction as it is impossible to separate patient satisfaction from other elements of care. Patients and families are looking at all aspects of care from the hospital environment, ease of use, perceived quality of care, and the relationships with the healthcare team, and among members of that team. As shown in Fig. 10.2, service is only as good as the weakest link in the chain; therefore, physicians need to pay close attention to supporting and training all team members. They should aim to hire competent people who are willing to learn and can follow agreed upon standards. Exam rooms need to be clean with comfortable furniture to seat patients and accommodate family members or friends.

Fig. 10.2 Satisfaction is interwined with other elements of care

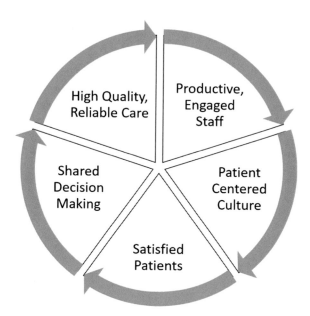

Limitations to Measuring Patient Satisfaction

As patient satisfaction is increasingly tied to reimbursement and individual physician compensation and scores are publicly reported, it is important to consider if adjustment of scores is warranted based on physician characteristics, such as gender, race, or practice setting. Factors out of an individual provider's control including patients' gender role expectations, the race and gender of the treating physician, and nonverbal behaviors may play an important role in patient satisfaction. An evaluation of women treated by an outpatient gynecologist found that female gynecologists were 47% less likely to receive a top box score on the HCAHPS survey likelihood to recommend physician compared with male gynecologists after adjusting for the health care environment [5]. In contrast, a study of psychiatrists in Norway found female physicians had more satisfied inpatients and patients in the emergency department compared with male physicians, while no differences were identified in the outpatient setting [6]. A study of nonverbal behavior in general practitioners with university students as analog patients demonstrated satisfaction was higher when female physicians practiced in a professional setting (white coat, medical-looking exam room) and behaved in line with gender stereotypes (more forward lean, more gazing, softer voice) [13]. Patients have also been found to have a preference for the care setting and how physicians dress and patient preferences varied across specialties and gender [14]. An analysis of a six hospital health system demonstrated no association between physician age, gender, or training and satisfaction; however, physician race was associated with patient satisfaction with South Asian, East Asian, and Black American physicians receiving significantly lower satisfaction scores as compared with White American physicians [7]. International medical graduates have also been found to be significantly less likely to receive a top box score across 10 HCAHPS survey questions [8]. Patients' perception of room cleanliness is often lower when the physician they saw is a minority physician compared to white physicians, even if they all practiced using the very same rooms. Going forward, it will be imperative to better understand the role of non-modifiable provider characteristics and bias in healthcare in driving patient satisfaction given the implications on public reporting, reimbursement, and compensation.

Future of Patient Satisfaction

In addition to measuring and responding to patient satisfaction, healthcare organizations and physicians will need to evaluate drivers of patient satisfaction including patient-centered care, employee engagement, patient education, reliability and coordination of care. Hospitals can learn from high-performing industries such as aviation, manufacturing, construction, and finance to improve patient safety and reliability. They can also learn how to optimize patient experience from service industry leaders such as Disney, where the pervasive culture is focused on the guest experience.

While incorporating patient satisfaction scores into hospital reimbursement schema has placed an added emphasis on patient satisfaction, other measures of patient-centered care such as PROMs are likely to play an important role in the future. PROMs measure procedure-specific outcomes that are important to patients and providers, as opposed to overall satisfaction measure used in other surveys. Therefore, PROMs provide a more granular view of the patient's physical, emotional, and psychosocial responses to treatment. New regulation and demands by patient and payers are likely to increase transparency in reporting of all outcomes allowing consumers to compare hospitals and leading to more focus by providers and hospitals on efforts to improve outcomes and patient experience.

In order to make a measurable difference in patient satisfaction, the organization and providers have to genuinely want to provide high-quality, patient-centered care. If the focus is solely on raising satisfaction scores or reimbursement, it will be difficult to change the institutional culture and patient satisfaction scores. The most reliable way to produce highly satisfied patients and families is with a pervasive culture of quality and safety, sincere efforts to engage patients and families, and providing the care in an environment that we would want for our own family. The majority of adults are now using social media with approximately half of seniors now using Facebook. There are ample venues to share experiences at this time from Twitter to Yelp! to SnapChat to blogs and Facebook posts. While these tools may not have a direct relationship with objective data of care quality, or even with the results of standard surveys such as HCAHPS, hospitals and physicians are paying greater attention to online postings and seeking help from media experts to monitor and respond to patient comments. Soon the days of post-discharge surveys will be in the distant past and patients will be able to express their opinions on an ongoing basis using handheld devices, apps, or computers to provide feedback to physicians and their team. Physicians will receive the data in real time, giving them the opportunity to respond to patient concerns as they arise. The collective timely feedback from patients in a hospital, if appropriately monitored, can be a very useful barometer to gauge how well a given unit is doing in meeting patients' needs and where help needs to be dispatched to attend to any deficiency. This will no doubt allow for greater participation of patients and their family in their care and should further improve patient satisfaction with the care they receive.

Ways to improve patient satisfaction
Compassionate care
Culture of patient-centered care
Clear, open communication
Shared decision making
Team work amongst multi-disciplinary team
Supportive and comfortable hospital environment.

References

1. Stefl ME. To err is human: building a safer health system in 1999. Front Health Serv Manage. 2001;18(1):1–2.
2. Tevis SE, Schmocker RK, Kennedy GD. Can patients reliably identify safe, high quality care? J Hosp Adm. 2014;3(5):150–60.
3. HCAHPS Survey.
4. Hospital compare. www.medicare.gov/hospitalcompare/search.html.
5. Rogo-Gupta LJ, et al. Physician gender is associated with press ganey patient satisfaction scores in outpatient gynecology. Womens Health Issues. 2018;28(3):281–5.
6. Hall JA, Gulbrandsen P, Dahl FA. Physician gender, physician patient-centered behavior, and patient satisfaction: a study in three practice settings within a hospital. Patient Educ Couns. 2014;95(3):313–8.
7. Martinez KA, et al. The association between physician race/ethnicity and patient satisfaction: an exploration in direct to consumer telemedicine. J Gen Intern Med. 2020;35(9):2600–6.
8. Engelhardt KE, et al. Physician characteristics associated with patient experience scores: implications for adjusting public reporting of individual physician scores. BMJ Qual Saf. 2019;28(5):412–5.
9. Kaye DR, et al. Association between patient satisfaction and short-term outcomes after major cancer surgery. Ann Surg Oncol. 2017;24(12):3486–93.
10. Schmocker RK, et al. Understanding the determinants of patient satisfaction with surgical care using the consumer assessment of healthcare providers and systems surgical care survey (S-CAHPS). Surgery. 2015;158(6):1724–33.
11. Shirk JD, et al. Patient experience and quality of urologic cancer surgery in US hospitals. Cancer. 2016;122(16):2571–8.
12. Balik B. Achieving an exceptional patient and family experience of outpatient care. IHI Innovation Series white paper. 2011.
13. Mast MS, et al. Physician gender affects how physician nonverbal behavior is related to patient satisfaction. Med Care. 2008;46(12):1212–8.
14. Petrilli CM, et al. Understanding patient preference for physician attire: a cross-sectional observational study of 10 academic medical centres in the USA. BMJ Open. 2018;8(5): e021239.

Chapter 11
Managing the Operating Room

David F. Jarrard

Introduction

Running an efficient operating schedule is a major part of a clinical urologist's practice. The operating room is one of the most costly areas in the medical system. A single surgical procedure can require many hours from physicians, assistants, and nurses. The Agency for Healthcare Research and Quality found that hospitalizations that involved surgery accounted for 48% of hospital costs. Thus, surgeon efficiency in the operating room not only improves the financial bottom line for the hospital, but also expands free time for the urologist to pursue administrative, academic, fitness, and family pursuits.

An early advocate of time management, Benjamin Franklin emphasized in his essay entitled '*The Way to Wealth*' some of the important themes for efficiency including "Time is money," and "Don't leave until tomorrow what you can do today". Efficiency and time management skills are rarely taught in medical school or residencies and gaining this knowledge is largely left to be learned through trial and error. Although there is an overabundance of literature on time management strategies in the corporate and industrial world, little has been written for physicians and more specifically surgeons. The increasing demand on physician's time by electronic medical records, documentation and billing can generate increased physician frustration and burnout.

This chapter will address themes to improve efficiency and quality in the peri- and intraoperative environment. Decreasing operative case time may have other

D. F. Jarrard (✉)
Department of Urology, University of Wisconsin School of Medicine and Public Health, 7037, Wisconsin Institutes of Medical Research, 1111 Highland Avenue, Madison, WI 53792, USA
e-mail: jarrard@urology.wisc.edu

University of Wisconsin Carbone Cancer Center, 600 Highland Ave, Madison, WI 53705, USA

© The Author(s), under exclusive license to Springer Nature Switzerland AG 2022   99
S. Y. Nakada and S. R. Patel (eds.), *Navigating Organized Urology*,
https://doi.org/10.1007/978-3-031-05540-9_11

benefits including improved outcomes for the patient. For multiple procedures, shorter operative time (adjusted for case complexity and other factors) is associated with decreased infection rates and superior surgical outcomes [1–3]. Based on these analyses of large databases, some authors have proposed operative time be considered as an individual quality metric, and an alternative to case volume [1]. Regardless, there are many compelling reasons to run an efficient operating room and nearly all of them require the attention of the surgeon in setting up the processes for well-organized care. Metrics for the urologist to consider in an effort to improve efficiency include first case start times, case times, turnover times and patient complications and outcomes.

Navigating the Operating Room: Best Practices

Preoperative holding. Meeting the patient and the family in the preoperative area is a critical component of a successful operating room. Conducting a review to update yourself on any important changes in the patient's past medical conditions, surgical history, and recent events pertaining to the disease. Review the consent and mark the affected side on the patient. Briefly review the planned course of action highlighting any decisions that might be encountered during the case. For example, if extensive, unrecognized metastatic disease is present this may require a change in operative plan. Outline the planned course of hospitalization. At the end of the conversation, ask the patient (and attendant family) if they have any further questions. Discuss with the family plans for communication during and after the operation.

This preoperative meeting is greatly facilitated by preoperative education done during the prior clinic meeting or at some point prior to the surgery date. In addition to the surgeon outlining the procedure, complications and expected outcomes, meeting with nursing to outline the details on preoperative preparation can improve patient satisfaction. We have also employed a series of educational videos for common urologic procedures (e.g., stone treatment, TURP, radical prostatectomy) that further educate the patient. These approaches increase knowledge, provide reassurance and multiple opportunities for the patient to ask questions. This results in an efficient, smoother hospital course. Clearly, if an emergent procedure, this transfer of information needs to be compressed and requires more time on the day of the procedure.

Reviewing the case and equipment with staff. Take a few minutes before the patient enters the operative theater to orient the team to the case including positioning, length of time, potential blood loss, and any unusual aspects. Reviewing the equipment needed or potentially needed, the sutures required, and other aspects will help avoid confusion and ultimately improve patient safety, quality of care and team satisfaction. Make certain the required films are present and displayed in the operating room.

<u>Visualization</u>. The role of preparation and visualization *prior to the operation* is an important tool for the newer surgeon and for cases that are more complex. Picturing the case steps, possible decision points and progression of the case helps with set up, speed of the operation, and increases the likelihood of a successful outcome. Reviewing one's notes or literature on complex cases encountered and their operative approach can help with this process.

Of note, tardiness in the operating room is one of the worst sins a surgeon can commit. A morning case that begins 30 min late has repercussions for the entire day. Additionally, it undermines the motivation and efficiency of the staff and results in loss of team cohesion.

<u>Time-out</u>. The time-out is an important safety and efficiency step just prior to the operation. A time-out is a universal patient safety protocol performed by the surgical team to prevent errors in surgery. In the operating room before anesthesia is initiated the team and the patient review the correct patient, side and type of surgery, available equipment, medications, and fire safety. A time-out involves the surgeons, anesthesia providers, circulating nurses, operating room technicians, students, and other members present in the operating room. If multiple procedures by different teams will be performed, a time-out needs to be reviewed for each procedure individually.

<u>Progression through the case</u>. Efficient use of time in the operating room is important. Operating room time is expensive, and this charge begins the minute the patient enters the operating room theater. The lead surgeon can set the tone for efficient use of this time by employing several techniques. Paying attention to all aspects of the procedure from checking positioning to prepping the patient with antibacterial solution. If the staff is busy with other aspects of the setup, pitching in and helping shave and prepare the patient emphasizes the importance of efficiency and is a positive message to the team.

During progression of the case, verbally letting the scrub assistant know what is needed for the next step (or steps) before reaching that point can save 10–15 s or more at numerous points, all of which adds up to time saved over a longer case. Not having to wait for a suture, a drain or other equipment also improves the 'rhythm' of the case and helps decrease stress on the assistants and circulating staff. Multiple studies have shown the most frequent disruptors in operative cases are equipment-related and miscommunication and/or coordination [4, 5].

<u>Team building</u>. Creating a culture of open communication among the team is important for efficiency and above all patient safety. Identifying these problems ahead of time can help surgeons and their teams avoid a time-consuming setback in the middle of an operation. Banter regarding non-case related issues is important in the operating room during less busy critical or stressful periods. This can reinforce collegiality and make the operating a more pleasant environment especially for those members of the team who are required to be there every day. Similarly, music can help as a pleasant distractor for the staff provided it does not interfere with communication or concentration.

Microbreaks. Archival literature has demonstrated ergonomic risks to surgeons in the operating room. One method used in other industries to mitigate these problems is the incorporation of microbreaks. In surgery, these can consist of 1.5–2 min exercises performed intraoperatively within the sterile field or at the console at medically convenient 20–40 min intervals throughout each case over the surgical day. These targeted sets of exercises focus on the neck, back, shoulders, hands, and lower extremities. Benefits include an improvement in mental focus, better physical performance, and a reduction in short-term and long-term pain without significantly altering operative duration [6]. Encouraging the participation of all members of the operative team in these exercises may reduce stress, and improve team performance.

Resident teaching. Teaching in the operating room affects efficiency and operative time, but remains a critical part of medical care. In a recent study at a major academic center, roughly half of the operative case time was spent teaching [7]. Directing, commenting, and informing behaviors, and responding to questions and/ or comments comprised the most common teaching methods. Changes in the approach and amount of teaching can vary based on several factors including the complexity of the case, the schedule, and the direct physical control the attending surgeon has at any one time.

Teaching laparoscopic/robotic and open surgical cases may require different approaches. With open cases, the resident may be provided with more flexibility since the primary surgeon has more direct, hands-on control over the case, physically assisting the resident during each step. Alternatively, this is more difficult with minimally invasive cases. A useful teaching approach that impacts operative time minimally and can be employed with similar cases done multiple times in a day or week (e.g., robotic prostatectomy) is a division of the operation into segments based on skill level. One example with robotic prostatectomy divides the case into robotic docking and port placement, prostate exposure, bladder neck dissection, nerve sparing and apical dissection, and urethral anastomosis. Allowing the resident to repeatedly perform the same segment(s) leads to quicker progression, satisfaction and ultimately autonomy, while minimizing the impact on overall case time.

Completing the case. As the operative procedure is finishing and before the wound is closed, taking a few minutes to have the operative team perform a review is important for safety and efficiency. Confirming the procedure, and reviewing accurate specimen labeling, wound classification, blood loss, complications, surgical sponge count and any key patient concerns for recovery and management are part of this debrief.

Room turnover. Lengthy turnovers are a source of significant dissatisfaction among surgeons, who see turnovers as lost operative time. Are there aspects that the surgeon can help with? Making certain that the next case is consented and reviewed including alerting the operative team to any special requirements prevents delays. Setting expectations can assist to a point, but may have unintended consequences related to quality. The best approach is to be supportive and available should any issues arise.

Complications and outcomes. Tracking untoward events and complicating factors are critical in the pursuit of efficiency for the surgeon. These include both perioperative and postoperative events. From the surgeon standpoint, providing consistency of service is important for patients, hospitals, and operating rooms. This consistency also extends to other team members including anaesthesia, nursing, and other staff. It is important for the surgeon to monitor his or her results with regard to infection, bleeding, hospital stay as well as readmission rate. Starting in 2010 Medicare began requiring ambulatory surgery centers (ASCs) to report surgical complications 30 days after the procedure and one year afterwards for implants. Similarly, readmission within 30 days is tracked for procedures requiring inpatient admission. Longer-term outcomes are also important and require monitoring by the urologist including recurrence, failure, and other commonly reported case features. This feedback can identify areas of deficiency and ultimately result in improved patient care and consistency.

Other components to navigate. In the modern hospital system, new surgeons should be aware that the traditional method of basing block time on each individual surgeons' potential utilization rates has evolved to the more frequently based approach based on under- and overutilization. If the surgeon is unable to utilize time for whatever reason, block releases are one way for operating room managers to improve efficiency. Utilizing block time to its greatest potential (>80%) is an aspect that many hospitals and surgery centers demand.

Efficiency in the operating room also involves using resources wisely. Checking supply costs against national averages gives the individual surgeon information on how your costs compare to national averages. Learning from colleagues that generate less cost can help improve this metric. Standardization of certain equipment may meet with some initial surgeon resistance, but ultimately may lead to cost savings due to efficiencies of scale, and reduced waste due to product expiration.

Some centers have also begun tracking the cost of labor per case to identify surgeons who are taking longer to complete a standard case. This includes using more staff per case or using more expensive staff for example registered nurses instead of technicians. This metric can help explain variance between surgeons and provides opportunities for process improvement.

Conflict invariably arises in the operating room where patient responsibility is shared and disagreements arise due to personal differences, informational deficiency, role incompatibility, and environmental stress [8]. Roughly 20% of the physician executive's time was spent in dealing with these conflicts [9]. A professional relationship is required between two or more physicians, in order to provide care in a safe and appropriate manner. For example, postponement or cancelation of a planned surgical procedure by anesthesia due to poorly controlled systemic diseases or other factors occurs frequently from 2 to 14% in some studies [10]. As a surgeon, it is critical to work to resolve these issues with the realization that patient safety and care is and should be the primary driving force. Similarly, conflict between the surgeon and nursing or other support staff may arise and can lead to stress and patient safety issues. If this situation arises, it is important to step back in order to avoid escalating the situation and look for a neutral mediator (e.g., anesthesiologist, staff surgeon leader, nursing supervisor) to help resolve the situation. This additional view can help to depersonalize the issues, defuse tensions, and find a solution. The reaffirmation of the common goal of patient care and the recognition of the legitimate differences can often work toward resolving differences.

COVID-19. "May you live in interesting times." This curse certainly applies to the COVID-19 pandemic and its effects on American and other health care systems. It has negatively impacted our ability to efficiently organize and run the operating room. The pandemic has added burdens and stress to surgeons regarding triaging cases given limited resources, as well as preoperative screening and requirements for virus testing. During the operative phase, health teams are at high risk of virus transmission and safety measures employing N95 masks, in addition to droplet PPE (gown, gloves, eye protection) remain additional challenges. In the postoperative phase, there are added recommendations for managing operating theaters and patient transfers. Throughout, maintaining the safety and well-being of the operative team should be of paramount importance to the attending surgeon. By approaching new and evolving recommendations with a positive mind, and demonstrating flexibility these new aspects can be incorporated into the efficient and well-run operating room.

Conclusions

Running an efficient operating room has a number of advantages including cost, reduced stress, and additional time. Operating room efficiency directly reflects on the triple aim of patient care including lower cost, outstanding care, and patient safety. By establishing these behaviors and expectations early, these practices will pay dividends in productivity and satisfaction for years to come.

Key Points

- Be early and present in the operating room.
- Spend time orienting the staff to the case and checking equipment
- During the case, be proactive, communicative, and forward thinking.
- Tracking your complications and outcomes and comparing these to national metrics are important to efficiency and quality.
- Setting up the expectations of efficiency and quality will pay dividends in terms of more time for your career, leisure, and family as well as better patient care.

References

1. Garnett G, Wilkens L, Limm W, Wong L. Operative time as a measure of quality in pancreaticoduodenectomy: is faster better? A retrospective review using the ACS NSQIP Database. Surg Sci. 2015;6:418–26.
2. Jackson TD, Wannares JJ, Lancaster RT, Rattner DW, Hutter MM. Does speed matter? The impact of operative time on outcome in laparoscopic surgery. Surg Endosc. 2011;25:2288–95.
3. Campbell DA Jr, et al. Surgical site infection prevention: the importance of operative duration and blood transfusion–results of the first American College of Surgeons-National Surgical Quality Improvement Program Best Practices Initiative. J Am Coll Surg. 2008;207:810–20.
4. Shouhed D, et al. Flow disruptions during trauma care. World J Surg. 2014;38:314–21.
5. Cohen TN, et al. Identifying workflow disruptions in the cardiovascular operating room. Anaesthesia. 2016;71:948–54.
6. Hallbeck MS, et al. The impact of intraoperative microbreaks with exercises on surgeons: a multi-center cohort study. Appl Ergon. 2017;64:334–41.
7. Glarner CE, et al. Resident training in a teaching hospital: how do attendings teach in the real operative environment? Am J Surg. 2017;214:141–6.
8. Lipcamon JD, Mainwaring BA. Conflict resolution in healthcare management. Radiol Manage. 2004;26:48–51.
9. Katz JD. Conflict and its resolution in the operating room. J Clin Anesth. 2007;19:152–8.
10. van Klei WA, et al. The effect of outpatient preoperative evaluation of hospital inpatients on cancellation of surgery and length of hospital stay. Anesth Analg. 2002;94:644–9.

Chapter 12
Enhancing and Promoting Your Office Urology Practice: Future Trends in Technology

David Mobley and Neil Baum

As a result of the recent COVID-19 pandemic in 2020/2021, decreasing patient visits, decreasing procedures/surgery, lowered reimbursements, and rising overhead costs, doctors are looking for methods and techniques to become more efficient and more productive. Just a few decades ago, the only opportunity to promote our practices was to announce our practice in the local newspaper and include our address and phone number. Anything beyond that announcement was considered inappropriate and unethical. Fortunately, we have come a long way since the 1970s and have discovered methods of effective and ethical practice promotion. This chapter will discuss future trends in medical marking in the 2020s.

Urologists today are challenged like no other time in our glorious history. Trends are taking place to move surgical patients from the operating room to the office setting using minimally invasive surgery instead of in-hospital procedures. There is a continuous trend of moving from open surgery to robotic and laparoscopic surgery. There is movement from a solo practice to large group practices and younger urologists are being employed by hospitals instead of joining groups or starting in solo practice. There is also a trend for urologists to become involved in the business of medicine as many more are pursuing combined MD and MBA degrees [1]. The aging baby boomers will have increasing medical problems requiring our attention, and there will be additional demands upon physicians, particularly urologists. With physicians retiring at an earlier age and with inadequate replacements to accommodate the increased number of patients, there are going to be serious time challenges for physicians. The take-home message is that urologists are going to be more efficient and more productive in order to adapt to the future. One opportunity for all urologists is to improve their efficiency by treating various urologic diseases

D. Mobley
Clinical Urology, Weill Cornell Medicine, Houston, TX, USA

N. Baum (✉)
Professor of Clinical Urology, Tulane Medical School, New Orleans, LA, USA
e-mail: doctorwhiz@gmail.com

© The Author(s), under exclusive license to Springer Nature Switzerland AG 2022
S. Y. Nakada and S. R. Patel (eds.), *Navigating Organized Urology*,
https://doi.org/10.1007/978-3-031-05540-9_12

and conditions in the office instead of in the hospital. This chapter will discuss the advantages to patients, physicians, and insurance companies of becoming more productive by seeing more patients in an efficient manner and doing more procedures in the office than previously could only be done in the hospital operating room. This chapter will discuss the patient cycle from initial contact to after they leave the practice and become raving fans. We will also provide our opinions regarding technology in contemporary urologic practice and what the future may hold.

Before the Patient Enters the Practice

The interaction of the patient with the practice begins long before the physician is eyeball to eyeball with the patient. It usually starts with the telephone. The individual who answers your telephone is the lifeline of your practice. Far too often office managers delegate the job of answering the telephones to the employee with the least amount of training and the lowest salary. A new patient's initial telephone call is the first interaction between the patient and your practice. During that telephone interaction, your practice has a golden opportunity to create a positive first impression on the caller. If you (or your office ambassador, the receptionist) fail to create a positive impression, the patient may form a negative opinion toward you and your practice even before opening the door of your office to meet you or your staff. Our take-home message: you only get one chance to create a first impression.

Next, you want the receptionist to direct the patient to the practice's website. If possible, the receptionist identifies the reason for the visit to the urologist. The well-informed and knowledgeable receptionist directs the caller to a page that has educational material pertinent to the reason for their visit to the urologist. For example, if the patient is requesting an appointment for an evaluation of an elevated PSA level, the receptionist can direct the patient to information on the practice website about PSA elevation and what are the tests and procedures that might be done to evaluate the rise in the PSA. Likewise, it is valuable to have information on your website about common urologic conditions and treatments such as BPH, epididymitis, and treatment for localized prostate cancer.

In order to become more efficient, the patient should complete their demographic information and complete a health questionnaire before they come to the office. These forms should be on the website and can be submitted electronically or printed from the website and the hard copy brought with the patient to the office and then scanned into the patient's EMR. Completing these documents prior to the first visit avoids the patient waiting in the reception area for 20–30 min completing this information prior to their visit. Patients are told that this will expedite their visit if they complete this information prior to the visit. Patients should also be told to bring a list of all of their medications including any over-the-counter pills or supplements that they are using.

The patients are also informed that the visit will be more efficient and meaningful if they bring copies of their lab work or results of any tests or procedures. For example, if they have had previous blood tests, imaging studies, or pathology reports, these should be brought by the patient at the time of their visit. This avoids having reports sent to the office and the reports not being able to be easily located, or the situation where the urology office calls another office to receive a copy of a report which usually necessitates a signed request, retrieval of the report, and the time it takes to FAX the report to the urology office. All of which can significantly delay the visit and result in a significant loss of efficiency, as well as some unnecessary frustration for the patient and physician. Another simple suggestion is for the receptionist to tell the patient that a urine specimen will be necessary at the time of the first visit. The patients should be informed about consuming ample volumes of fluids before they come to the office and the patient is to inform the front desk that they are ready to provide a specimen upon arrival. The receptionist informs the patient of an estimate of how long the first visit might take and what will be done during that visit. For example, if a man is being evaluated for an enlarged prostate gland, then he might be told that he will be requested to do a flow rate, a bladder ultrasound, and possibly a cystoscopy. He then should be told that the procedures are explained on the website and that he should read about the tests so he is ready to have the tests upon arrival in the office.

These are simple steps that can be easily accomplished by any urology practice resulting in a significant improvement in practice efficiency. Now a new patient can begin the process of becoming a part of the practice even before they enter the practice. These few steps make it easy for the patient and staff, and improve the efficiency and productivity of the practice, allowing the urologist to see more patients while still providing the same level of care.

When the Patient has Arrived in Your Practice

The patient arrived and has already provided the demographic information and the health questionnaire before they come to the office, so the patient has been taken to the examination room. The physician should meet the patient and have a 1–2 min discussion about some areas outside of their medical/urologic concerns, i.e., what kind of work do you do, where do you live, and who referred you to our practice? These are the questions that endear the patient to the urologist without discussions specific to the urologic problem.

To enhance efficiency, the urologist may use a scribe to take the history of the present illness, the review of systems, and the past medical history. One of the most effective methods to enhance the efficiency of almost any practice is to make use of a scribe. A scribe is a staff member who shadows a physician and takes notes either on the chart, or better yet, on the computer, thus freeing the physician to have more eye-to-eye contact with the patient.

How Does the Scribe Work?

The scribe interacts with a new patient after the doctor introduces him/herself to the patient. The scribe then takes the history of the present illness, records the past medical history, and the review of systems. The scribe then presents the HOPI to the physician and then accompanies the physician into the room. At this point, the physician is likely to ask a few additional questions or probe any aspects of the HOPI that are not clear or need a more in-depth questioning. The physician conducts the physical examination, then the scribe records the positive findings in the chart or the EMR. At this juncture, the urologist can have a discussion with the patient regarding the diagnosis and the plan of management with the patient and the scribe records the doctor's plan of action. The physician can then answer any questions the patient may have and the scribe can give the chart or the computer to the nurse who will make the necessary arrangements for any lab tests, studies, or surgeries, provide the patient with sample medications and written instructions for the use of the medications, provide pertinent educational materials, and make the follow-up appointments. While the nurse is taking care of one patient, the scribe has moved to the next patient, staying one patient ahead of the physician.

Advantages of the Scribe

Most of all, your scribe improves the efficiency of the practice. You are now able to be eye-to-eye with the patient and focus on communicating with the patient instead of writing or using the computer. As a result of using the scribe, you are able to see 5–6 additional patients each full day in the office. Also, coding may move from a previous level 2–3 to level 4–5 as the scribe is more thorough in conducting the review of systems, past medical history, and recording the fine nuances of the physical examination that are often neglected to document, such as a neurologic and dermatologic examination.

The disadvantages of having a scribe are cost, time to train the scribe, and the changing of habits from you doing the writing in the chart or working the computers to allowing someone else to do it for you. In the beginning, this can be frustrating, but when you see how efficient you become, you will enjoy the luxury of having a scribe. As a matter of fact, when the scribe is absent or on vacation and you have to use the computer, you clearly realize how invaluable your scribe is and how effective the technique is to enhance your practice.

We have also found the use of templates that will enable the scribe to ask all of the appropriate questions to create a thorough chief complaint. We are attaching samples of the templates for erectile dysfunction and BPH at the end of this chapter.

Getting Started

First, decide if you need a scribe. If patients need to wait more than 4–6 weeks to make an appointment for a routine visit, then you have a backlog of patients, and a scribe will help you reduce that backlog. If your last patient is scheduled at 4 or 4:30 and you are not finished with patients until 5:30 or 6:00, a scribe may help improve the efficiency of your practice. If the majority of your codes are Level 3 or less, you may improve your productivity by having a scribe. Finally, if you have not yet moved to an EMR but are technophobic, then a scribe might be a natural segue to implementing the EMR.

No chapter on efficiency and productivity would be complete without mentioning the use of physician assistants (PA) and nurse practitioners (NP). PA/NP may play a crucial role in the future of healthcare because of the rising number of patients needing care, i.e., the aging of the baby boomer population with nearly 10,000 people turning 65 every day, and the pressing demands upon a urologist's time. Using PA/NP may decrease healthcare costs, enable faster delivery of care, and shorten wait times for patients. PA/NP spend time consulting with patients and reviewing lab tests, history, and chronic conditions. After the PA/NP presents the patient's condition to physicians, the PA/NP and the urologist collaborate to form a diagnostic and treatment plan. The physician then meets with patients to deliver the assessment and care instructions. This model has been successfully used and enables physicians to see more patients per day, while still providing quality care.

Using Videos to Educate Your Patients

Urologists, now more than ever before, will need to be more efficient in order to remain more productive. It was not but a few years ago that physicians saw low volumes of patients and were able to spend time educating patients about their medical condition and helping them understand the importance of being compliant. Now urologists are going to need to see larger volumes of patients and will be spending less time with each patient and will not have the luxury of lengthy explanations about their health and providing them with one-to-one educational discussions. Nowadays, patients are relying on the Internet and other sources such as social media to obtain medical information. As a result, patients are often less compliant and when compliance has been decreased, the outcomes are often less desirable.

In the recent past, the formula for practice productivity was low patient volumes, substantial reimbursements in a fee-for-service arrangement, and good doctor–patient relationships. Today with the Affordable Care Act, the situation is reversed: large patient volumes, decreased reimbursements for the same services that were performed a few years ago, and less time spent with each patient. In order to maintain productivity, urologists will be forced to see more patients at the same time as a few years ago. As a result of spending less time with patients, there is less opportunity to spend time educating patients. Patients may be less compliant because they have less information about their medical condition and this may portend a deterioration in patient outcomes.

With the use of videos, you can educate patients with exactly the message you want them to receive. This is far more effective and appreciated than videos distributed by pharmaceutical companies and vendors of equipment that you may use in your office and in the hospital. With regards to videos, we suggest that you select topics that you discuss with patients on a regular basis. If you have a discussion with patients about PSA elevation several times a day or week, this would be an appropriate topic for a video. We like to select topics that are of current interest to patients. Next, you will need to create a script. In most instances, the script can follow the format shown in Fig. 12.1. The script serves as a teleprompter by putting the bullet points into a PowerPoint presentation. The quality of the video created with the iPhone, or Android from Samsung, is excellent. The only other piece of equipment that we recommend is a flexible tripod to hold the iPhone. These are available on Amazon at http://www.amazon.com/dp/B017NA7V1U?psc=1 (Fig. 12.2). With the smartphone on the tripod attached to the computer and the PowerPoint program

Fig. 12.1 Sample of a script format

1. Definition of the procedure or test

2. How the procedure or test is performed

3. Patient preparation for the test or procedure

4. Expectations after the procedure or test

5. Risks and complications and their relative frequency

6. Alternatives of treatment

Fig. 12.2 Example of tripod that holds the smart phone for creating DIY videos

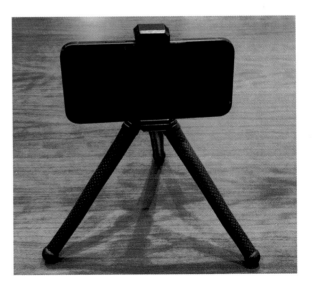

serving as your notes, you are ready to create a video. We suggest that videos be limited to 5–7 min as that is a reasonable attention span for most patients. Now the videos can be uploaded to your EMR or on separate computers in each of your examination rooms. Each video might end with the statement, "I hope you have found this video on <name of topic> helpful, and if you open the door at the end of the video, I will return to the exam room and provide you with a summary of the <topic> and will answer any questions you may have." We refer to this as the "sandwich" technique where the physician interacts with the patient first, performs the examination, followed by showing the video, and ending with the physician returning to the room to answer any questions that the patient may have about the topic.

Advantages of Creating Videos

When patients are watching the video, you can be seeing additional patients or perform brief office procedures. You can anticipate a 15–20% improvement in office efficiency by using educational videos. You can also find that patients will appreciate the education and the written summary that should accompany each video.

Videos and Medical–Legal Protection

Documentation is necessary in order to protect ourselves from litigation. It is possible using videos to demonstrate that the patient received information and education by documenting in the chart that the patient saw the video on a condition, procedure, or surgery. We suggest that you also include that all questions were answered before the patient left the office. To confirm that the patient *understood* the condition, the surgery, or the procedure, you can use a true/false questionnaire that the patient can answer after watching the video and include this in the chart. An example of a questionnaire that we use *after* the patient watches a video on vasectomy is shown in Fig. 12.3. This questionnaire and the results can be added to your medical records with a statement such as " <name of patient> watched a video

1. True or False. The ejaculate or fluid may contain sperm after two months or longer following a vasectomy.
2. True or False. Complications following a vasectomy include bleeding, infection, and\or pain.
3. True or False. Two semen analyses are necessary two months after a vasectomy to determine whether the vasectomy was successful or not.
4. True or False. A pregnancy may occur months or years after a successful vasectomy.

Fig. 12.3 Example of post video questionnaire on vasectomy

on the treatment of stress incontinence. The video discussed the procedure, risks, and complications, alternatives of treatment, including the option to have no treatment. She agrees to proceeding with a mid-urethral sling using synthetic mesh and understands the risks and complications associated with the use of mesh." We believe this makes the video an excellent form of medical–legal protection for the doctor and that the video enhances the informed consent process. Since the video is essentially a legal document, be certain that everything on the video is accurate and truly relates to your educational intention.

The marketing and promotion strategies of the past are not enough to promote practices in 2021 and beyond. The Internet is leveling the playing field in the area of medical knowledge. Several decades ago, the physician was the holder of the medical knowledge and patients came to physicians for his/her advice and knowledge. Today, a motivated patient with a computer and Internet access can learn as much about the pathophysiology and treatment of heart disease or any other condition as a physician. Physicians once viewed as the royal dispensers of specialized knowledge now see patients who have researched their medical condition and arrive with a file full of studies and a course of action from credible websites. Since it is possible that physicians do not have more information than patients anymore, it is our caring and compassion that will be important in helping patients follow our advice, be compliant in their follow-up, and improve their medical outcomes. Our new mantra should be "Computers (algorithms) will not replace us!" Physicians may find the following trends useful to market and promote their medical practice today and into the future.

Telemedicine

Perhaps the biggest game-changer for medical practices is telemedicine. The use of telemedicine has increased significantly since March 2020 when CMS waived requirements that limited telemedicine to distant site communication between patients and physicians and now includes all patients who have Medicare and Medicaid Medicare. In addition, CMS agreed to compensate physicians for virtual visits at the same rate as person-to-person visits. There has been a paradigm shift such that physicians are able to provide safe and effective care without the necessity of examining the patient. For example, we estimate that nearly 60% of urology patients can be managed using telemedicine. Many patients, especially millennials, will be looking for healthcare providers who offer virtual visits using telemedicine. Practices that do not offer to communicate with patients by way of telemedicine will probably lose patients.

Mobile Connections and Internet Searches

We know that many Americans use their smartphones to contact medical professionals. Therefore, it is imperative that your practice website is mobile-friendly in order to maintain current patients and attract new ones. It is also beneficial if your practice website is at the top of the results when someone does an Internet search for a medical practice. You can pay to have your name and the name of your practice at the top of the Google search. However, keywords, clever titles, and new content appearing on a regular basis can make your website attractive and ranked on the first page of search engines. Your rankings on the popular search engines will be enhanced if authoritative websites link to your website and reference you and your practice as an authority.

Social Media and Video Marketing

The effectiveness and influence of online social networking are undeniable, and it is no surprise that doctors are embracing it as a major component of their Internet marketing strategy. With leading social media sites, like Facebook, Twitter, and YouTube, it is never been easier to obtain or share content with your existing patients while increasing your visibility on the Internet and exposure to hundreds and even thousands of potential new patients. Millions of individuals gather online to network with other people and to acquire and share first-hand information and experiences about a number of topics, including the choice of a physician. Video marketing has been gaining a lot of steam on social media, especially with regard to healthcare companies. It is one of the healthcare marketing trends that is generating the highest levels of engagement. A majority of the public prefers watching videos about content rather than reading about it. Because healthcare is not an attention-grabbing topic on its own, video marketing can help create interest for your practice's services. When done well, videos can help attract and hold the attention of viewers and improve your reach. Short, content-rich videos of less than 2 min are the most effective. Videos can focus on the topics on which you differentiate yourself and your practice from others in the area. Another effective type of video for healthcare marketing is testimonials from existing patients and staff, which help build trust and credibility with current and potential patients.

If a picture is worth a thousand words, a video is probably worth 10,000 + words!

Psychographic Marketing

Demographic information, such as age, gender, race, address, and occupation, can be a starting point for targeting new patients, but it does not shed light on these potential patients' attitudes and mindset. Demographics explain "who" your patient is; psychographics explain "why." Psychographic information includes your potential patients' habits, hobbies, health-related experiences, and values—information you need to promote your services to a particular segment of the population. To reach ideal patients you must know what and who they value most, where they look for their medical information, and what content appeals to them. With that information, you can target specific messages about your areas of interest or expertise.

Cybersecurity

Cybersecurity is also a consideration in the digital marketing of the healthcare practice. Healthcare faces greater cyber risks than other sectors because of inherent weaknesses in its security posture. Many providers think that they are capable of defending themselves from cyberattacks, but that is folly. The healthcare sector is an attractive target for cyberattacks for two simple reasons: It is a rich source of valuable data, and it is a soft target [2]. Cybersecurity is not just about protecting data; it is fundamental for maintaining the safety, privacy, and trust of our patients. Effective cybersecurity must become an integral part of every medical practice.

Shifting from Illness to Wellness

Nearly 18% of the U.S. GDP is spent on healthcare—estimated at $3 T per annum —some suggest that $1T is wasted on duplicated tests, services, and defensive medicine [3].

Unfortunately, a huge gap exists between spending and outcomes. In fact, Americans lag near the bottom when it comes to health outcomes among wealthy countries [4]. One problem is that today's healthcare system focuses almost exclusively on responding to symptoms and illnesses. In the United States, we spend 97% of our healthcare resources on *disease* care [5]. But another vision for healthcare is emerging—one that is focused on *wellness* rather than illness. One that is proactive instead of reactive. One that focuses on population health rather than managing just a single patient. Within the past decade, big data, analytics, and social networks, as well as advances in technologies such as wearable health-tracking devices, are giving us the ability to learn more about wellness. That is the premise behind scientific wellness, which starts with a systems approach to analyzing highly specialized large data sets of individual human biomarkers such as genes, proteins, and microbiomes, combined with personalized health coaching to influence the health of our nation. Just as the Hubble Telescope provided a new view into the universe, personal, dense, dynamic data sets will be transformational for providing new insights into both human biology and disease [6]. This approach can help us better understand the genetic and environmental factors that determine our health status. Over time, this will enable us to identify the earliest transitions from wellness to disease, which is the key to both predictive and preventive care for individuals.

Precision Medicine and Precision Marketing

With an emphasis on personalized medicine, patients expect to be cared for to meet their individual needs. In addition to personalized medicine, we suggest you consider personalizing marketing to ensure the right patients are receiving the right messages. We recommend that the same theory of precision medicine be applied to the practice's healthcare marketing efforts.

"Dr. Alexa" Will See You Now

Alexa, Amazon's virtual assistant, is primed to perform healthcare-related tasks. "She" can track blood glucose levels, describe symptoms, access post-surgical care instructions, monitor home prescription deliveries, and make same-day appointments at the nearest urgent care center. Alexa can look at a picture of a wound and give advice if additional care is needed.

Alexa can also assist with your insurance claims. Liberty Mutual Insurance launched the first of its kind Alexa service that allows insurance buyers to navigate the policy purchase and management process purely by using their Amazon Echo [7].

A new Alexa skill will help furnish patients with all the detailed information about the hospital before they leave their homes. This will enable users to gain access to real-time information about the hospital, including:

- Parking information
- Visitor information
- Important contact information
- Bill payment information
- Directions to the hospital and the closest urgent care facility
- Info on how to view medical records
- Important things that you need to bring for your hospital stay.

Online Reputation Management

Physicians live and die by their reputations. We spend our entire medical careers polishing and protecting this status. The Internet has dramatically altered the way people gather information. It is sad but true that a single comment that takes only a few seconds for a patient to create and a single mouse-click to post on the Internet can be seen by thousands of visitors and ruin a physician's life-long reputation.

Never forget that your most precious asset is your reputation. Online physician reviews are positive 70–90% of the time [8].

However, physicians need to know the process of managing negative reviews. The best advice is to make sure you have many more positive reviews than negative reviews. That way an occasional negative review will not significantly detract from your online reputation.

Show Me the Money

A reasonable investment in marketing is 3–5% of the practice's gross revenues. However, marketers must be able to show that the money invested by a practice or a hospital demonstrates a return on the practice's investment. It is reasonable to ask a marketing firm about the expected increment in new patients or how the marketing firm plans to position the practice on the first page of Google.

Bottom Line: The genii is out of the bottle or the toothpaste is out of the tube and cannot be put back. We have an opportunity to harness the new trends in healthcare marketing. If you plan to be in practice for the foreseeable future, you will need to embrace a few of these suggestions and implement them into your practice. Most of them are easily accomplished with minimal expense and have been tested in other practices.

Erectile Dysfunction Template

ED Duration: ___weeks, ___months, ___ years
Intermittent: ___yes ___no; Nocturnal Erections: ___yes ___no
Partner specific: ___ yes ___no
Married: ___yes ___no   Divorced: ___yes ___no   Other: _____

IIEF or other Screening Tool:
Family History:_____
Libido: ___intact ___decreased ___treatment
Previous treatment: ___Viagra, ___Cialis, ___Levitra, ___Self-Injection Therapy, ___ VED,
                    ____Penile Prosthesis, ___Counseling
Testosterone: ____yes, ___no
Type of Testosterone: ____ Injection, ____ Pellet, ____Patch, ____Gel
Results of Treatment: _____ Successful, ____Not Successful
Co-Morbid Conditions: ____ Diabetes, ____Hypertension, ____Cholesterol ____CVD,
____OSA, ____Prostate Cancer, ____Sleep Apnea, _____UTI,
Smoking __yes, __no, ____Packs/Day, ____Chronic Back Pain, _____ Multiple Sclerosis
Urinary symptoms: _____
LUTS, ____AUA SS, ____Dysuria, _____Hematuria
Psychological evaluation: _____yes, _____no
Hx of premature ejaculation: _____yes, _____no
Penile curvature: _____yes, _____no, _____treatment
PSA in past year: _____yes, _____no, _____results ng\ml
Previous Surgery: _____
Current Medications: _____
Alcohol Consumption: ____yes, ___no, _____Drinks per week
Illicit drug use: marijuana: ____yes, ___no, Cocaine: ____yes, ___no Other:_____
PEx: Penis: _____plaque (cm), _____meatus, _____circumcised, _____length(cm)
   Testes:_____bilateral, _____absent R\L, _____ size (cm), ____tenderness
   Epididymis _____R _____L _____spermatocele
   DRE: estimated size (Gms), _____nodules _____location
   Neurologic exam: _____DTRs, _____sensation to light touch\pin prick
   Peripheral pulses: _____ Femoral R\L, _____D.Pedis R\L, _____P.Tibial R\L
Labs: T, Free\Total T; PSA, LH, FSH, Prolactin, TSH, Chol, BUN\Cr, LFTs, UA

Plan:
   Medications: _____
   Penile doppler:_____
   Lab tests ordered: _____
   Next appointment: _____ Other: _____

Time in Minutes: _____Pre-visit, _____Encounter, ____Post-visit, _____Total Time

Suggested E & M code _____

BPH Template

AUA SS: _____

LUTS: _____

Nocturia: _____number per night

Meds\Supplements: 5-alpha reductase inhibitors, alpha blockers,
        prostate supplements (saw palmetto, beta-sitosterol)

Fluid Consumption _____ estimated ounces\day

Caffeinated Beverages _____number per day

Sleep Hygiene _____ estimated hours per night

Previous Rx _____

Hematuria _____

Hx UTI, Dysuria _____

Prostate Infections _____

Previous Surgery _____

Cystoscopy: _____

DRE: size _____

        symmetry_____

        consistency _____

        tenderness _____

        rectal mass _____

        sphincter tone _____

UA\PSA _____

Flow Rate: _____cc\sec   volume voided_____

BUS\Residual Urine Volume _____ cc's

Prostate Ultrasound:

        width _____cm

        length_____cm

        estimated volume _____cc's

        symmetry _____

        calculi _____

        hypoechoic areas _____   location _____

Previous Treatment and Results: _____

Plan: _____

References

1. Russel J. Physicians who aren't good at business won't survive. Russel J, Washington Post, May 10, 2010.
2. KPMG. Health Care and Cybersecurity: Increasing Threats Require Increased Capabilities. KPMG; 2015.
3. Berwick DM, Hackbarth AD. Eliminating waste in US health care. JAMA. 2012;307 (14):1513–6.
4. Emanuel EJ, Gudbranson E, Van Parys J, Gørtz M, Helgeland J, Skinner J. Comparing health outcomes of privileged US citizens with those of average residents of other developed countries. JAMA Intern Med. 2021;181(3):339–44.
5. Martin AB, Hartman M, Lassman D, Catlin A. National Health Care Spending In 2019: Steady Growth For The Fourth Consecutive Year. Health Aff. 2020;40(1):1–11.
6. Hood L, Price, N. Turn healthcare right-side up: focus on wellness not disease. Psychology Today. March 19, 2018. www.psychologytoday.com/us/blog/the-social-brain/201803/turn-healthcare-right-side-focus-wellness-not-disease.
7. Insurance Journal. Liberty mutual giving consumers a voice in insurance via Amazon's Alexa. Insurance Journal. September 13, 2016.
8. Hall SD. Providers Responding to Yelp Reviews Must be Mindful of HIPAA. FierceHealthcare. www.fiercehealthcare.com/it/providers-responding-to-yelp-reviews-must-be-mindful-hipaa.

Chapter 13
Coding and Billing

David Paolone

Appropriate coding and billing for services performed are a critical endeavor for any successful urological practice. Unfortunately, very little formal education of the business of medicine is part of most urology residencies. Many residents and fellows may have some peripheral or informal exposure to the concepts of coding from attending physicians with a particular interest in this. However, many academic physicians themselves rely heavily on institutional support for obtaining proper reimbursement for work performed and have only a basic understanding of the elements of coding and coding themselves.

This chapter is not meant to be an exhaustive or detailed review of the nuances of coding and billing for all possible encounters in an outpatient urology clinic or for any number of inpatient and outpatient surgical procedures. Rather, the goal for the reader is to introduce some basic concepts in appropriate coding and billing, emphasize fundamentals regarding accuracy and honesty, and provide direction for ways of obtaining more advanced education in this topic and staying up to date with ever-changing rules and regulations [1–3].

Coding Basics

The most fundamental concept behind successful coding is to perform what is medically indicated and necessary for a particular patient with a given diagnosis, accurately document what is done in evaluating and treating the patient, and submit charges consistent with the above. Evaluation and management codes (E/M), surgical and procedure codes (CPT), modifying codes, and diagnostic codes (ICD-10)

D. Paolone (✉)

Department of Urology, University of Wisconsin School of Medicine and Public Health, Madison, WI 53715, USA

e-mail: DPaolone@uwhealth.org

© The Author(s), under exclusive license to Springer Nature Switzerland AG 2022   123

S. Y. Nakada and S. R. Patel (eds.), *Navigating Organized Urology*,

https://doi.org/10.1007/978-3-031-05540-9_13

are the language used to communicate the work done and the reason for doing it. The medical record must have supporting documentation for any work for which a physician seeks to obtain reimbursement. An overarching concept is that medical necessity trumps everything else when determination is made regarding what is permissible to be coded and billed for.

Evaluation and Management

Evaluation and management (E/M) services apply to patient evaluation in either the hospital or office setting. Medical history, physical examination, and medical decision making represent the three elements that have historically determined the appropriate level of service. The degree of complexity and detail for each of these elements would be used to calculate an appropriate level. Whether a patient is a new patient or established patient also determines how the appropriated code is selected. An established patient is one that has been seen by any provider within the practice in the previous three years. The Centers for Medicare and Medicaid Services (CMS) established documentation and coding requirements in 1995 and 1997, and these guidelines served as the foundation for proper billing and coding for over two decades. However, the guidelines for office and outpatient E/M codes were updated for 2021, with the goal to be to streamline the required documentation and reduce information included in the medical record that is not critical to patient care but rather only present for billing purposes.

For the history, the important elements required by the CMS 1995/1997 guidelines include history of present illness (including sub-elements of location, quality, severity, duration, timing, context, modifying factors, and associated signs and symptoms), review of systems (pertinent system being the genitourinary system with other systems reviewed as indicated for the chief complaint), and past medical, family, and social history. Obviously, these are all important elements to obtaining a thorough history for any patient and are critical to being able to make an appropriate differential diagnosis and determine a plan of care for further assessment and treatment. Any introductory class on physical examination and history taking in medical school should provide the foundation for a urologist to be able to quickly obtain this important information. A paper or online intake sheet is an efficient means of obtaining this information before the provider even sees the patient. The 2021 guidelines now simply require a medically appropriate history be documented as part of the encounter.

Physical examination includes a head to toe assessment of the patient from constitutional appearance and vital signs through a neurologic/psychiatric assessment. Obviously, the majority of the physical examination will likely be focused on the genitourinary and gastrointestinal(abdominal) systems. Prior to the implementation of the 2021 guidelines, the extent of the physical examination and the medical necessity of given elements of the exam for a particular diagnosis played a major role in selecting the correct E/M code for a patient encounter. However, another major difference between the 1995/1997 and 2021 guidelines is the need for documentation of only a medically appropriate physical examination, with the elements of the exam no longer playing a role in the code level selection.

Medical decision making consists of the number and complexity of problems or diagnoses addressed at the visit, the amount of data utilized to assess the symptoms (tests and radiological studies that are ordered and reviewed), and the level of risk of patient management for the given problem. Risk is determined by the stability or progression of a problem, the number and invasiveness of diagnostic procedures needed to assess the problem, and the potential complications of treatment options required to address the problem. A patient with a stable condition requiring only surveillance or oral medications will have a lower risk than a patient with a life-threatening condition requiring surgery. Two of the three above elements are needed to determine a level, and the lowest of the level of the two elements chosen equals the medical decision making level. A proper understanding of the terms and definitions involved in medical decision making is critical given that it is now the primary driver of E/M code determination beginning in 2021.

Probably the most efficient way for a urologist just starting out in practice to accurately determine the appropriate E/M code for patients being seen in clinic or in consultation at the hospital is to utilize a wall chart or pocket guide that summarizes all of the above elements with the point system to tally these elements and reach a given code. Once such chart is available from Relative Value Studies Incorporated and The PRS Network. With time, familiarity with the elements of the E/M coding system and repetition amongst commonly-seen diagnosis (new patient with hematuria, established patient with lower urinary tract symptoms due to benign prostatic hyperplasia, etc.) will allow appropriate coding to become second-nature and decrease reliance on such charts and guides. For new and unique patient encounters, however, a return to the basics may be invaluable in choosing the appropriate code.

An alternative to using the components outlined above also exists and may be more productive for a particular provider based on the nature of his/her practice. This alternative is to code utilizing time as the determinant for the level of service. The CMS 2021 guidelines have also changed the requirement for coding based on time. With the 1995/1997 guidelines, this was only an option if over 50% of the E/M encounter was spent on patient education and counseling regarding a particular problem or diagnoses, and documentation of the actual face-to-face time spent with the patient was critical to this type of coding. With the 2021 guidelines, the amount of time spent on the day of the visit spent on both face-to-face and non-face-to-face time is the factor that determines the appropriate coding level. Examples of non-face-to-face time activities that can be included in the time calculation are preparing for the visit by reviewing laboratory results and imaging studies, ordering medications, tests, or procedures, communicating with other healthcare professionals, documenting in the medical record, and otherwise coordinating care for the patient. The elements for history, physical examination, and medical decision making do not need to be reached for a particular level of coding if time is used, but honest measurement of time spent with the patient and the additional work for the visit on the day of the appointment is a must.

The explosion in the use of an electronic medical record (EMR) for documentation has had a profound impact on the practice of medicine and warrants a mention in the context of coding and billing. The use of templates, for example, may allow a provider to rapidly and efficiently complete documentation for an E/M visit and reduce the reliance on memory to make sure all elements of the history and examination are completed. Assigning an E/M code to each encounter can be quickly completed through the EMR, and this can speed up the process of billing to payers. However, use of the EMR is also fraught with the potential for abuse and fraud. Information imported from other sources without actually being obtained from or reviewed with the patient should not be counted in the elements of the history. Pre-population of physical exam findings in a template note risks inclusion of parts of a physical examination that were not actually performed. Cutting and pasting of elements of the history, physical examination, and assessment/plan from a past note into a current note must be avoided at all costs. Use of time references such a "yesterday" or "last week" that can lead to inaccuracies in a copied note rather than an actual date within an HPI make it obvious to an auditor that the note in question was not generated from a current discussion with the patient and therefore not acceptable for counting towards the level of service for a visit. Obviously, the use of an EMR will remain a critical tool for essentially every urologist entering practice, but one must balance its speed and convenience for documentation with the risk of profound challenges in accurately determining the appropriate level of service for an encounter based on what was actually discussed and performed.

Telemedicine

The coronavirus pandemic has had a profound effect on the delivery of medical care beginning in March of 2020. While telemedicine played a minor role in the routine delivery of care prior to the pandemic, the need to be able to administer medical evaluation and treatment in a safe manner for patients and providers created a significant shift towards this technology. Many practices have found a role for telemedicine as a long-term element to their overall services despite the easing of social distancing requirements. Each physician needs to find what works best with regard to which type of visits can be offered effectively as telemedicine visits. Routine follow-up visits for established patients where a physical exam is not likely to be required are a natural fit for this type of visit, and many patients have embraced this new approach to obtaining medical care. Whether new patient visits are suitable for this model, and which type of diagnoses are reasonable to see on a telemedicine platform are critical decisions for providers.

There are several practical considerations from a billing and coding standpoint that are relevant to telemedicine. It is critical to know the location of patients seen in this manner (which may be in a different state than the provider), and compliance with the licensing requirements regarding telemedicine for the state where both the patient and provider are located during the appointment is essential. There are dedicated E/M codes for scheduled appointments where the communication is done entirely via phone call, and these code levels are based entirely on time. For video visits, one utilizes the same E/M codes as those used for in-person visits. The CMS 2021 guidelines are particularly helpful for coding video visits given that an extensive physical examination is not necessarily required when coding is based on time or medical decision making. Utilizing a HIPAA compliant platform is another critical element to successful implementation of telemedicine for a practice.

Procedure Codes

A different language is utilized to accurately denote procedural work done in the operating room or the office setting. Current Procedural Terminology (CPT) codes represent a system for identifying interventions done and submitting a request to payers for payment of such services. These codes are maintained by the American Medical Association, and they are updated yearly. Obtaining the yearly book listing all such codes is critical to be able to accurately bill for surgical services provided. The CPT codes are five digit codes, and nearly every service provided by a urologist or other health care provide in other specialties will have its own individual CPT code. One must find the CPT code or codes that most closely resembles the procedure done. Unfortunately, there may be unique situations where a service is provided that does not necessarily fit into any currently available code. This represents one of the most challenging situations in the realm of coding and billing.

Bundling

A frequent occurrence in procedural coding is the fact that many procedures may be bundled into another CPT code for a more extensive or complicated procedure. This prevents overcharging for doing a procedure that is actually an essential component of a more complex procedure. For example, cystoscopy has its own unique CPT code. Transurethral resection of bladder tumor (TURBT) also has its own CPT code (in fact, there are several codes based on the size of the tumor being resected). When one performs a transurethral resection of a bladder tumor, a thorough cystoscopy is certainly performed first at the time of surgery to confirm the size and number of tumors. However, the CPT code for removal of the bladder tumor has cystoscopy bundled within it, and therefore, one would only submit the CPT code for TURBT rather than two separate CPT codes for both procedures. Examples of this situation are innumerable and must always be kept in mind when choosing the appropriate CPT code for services rendered. Adding to the confusion, there are certain circumstances when a procedure may be "unbundled" from another CPT code and billed for separately depending on a particular clinical scenario. The rules governing this change frequently, and thus it is essential that a urologist commit to continuing education regarding coding in order to prevent committing fraud or failing to achieve the maximum reimbursement for services provided.

Global Services

The concept of the global service is for a payer to combine all the payments for a particular service into one generalized payment to cover all the work necessary for that procedure. For example, rather than allowing a provider to bill individually for the preoperative visit, the surgery itself, and each individual post-operative encounter done in the hospital or the office, it may be more efficient and cost-effective for the payer to incorporate the reimbursement for the pre- and postoperative care into the charge for the surgery. Global periods can be 0 days, 10 days, or 90 days. The complexity of a surgical procedure will obviously determine into which of these global periods it will fall. For example, a uretero-scopy for a ureteral calculus has a 0 day global period. A urologist may therefore submit an E/M charge for a pre-operative visit, the CPT charge for the procedure itself, a CPT charge for a cystoscopy and stent removal a week after the procedure, and E/M charges for any office visits related to the calculus or other urological concerns any time after the primary surgical procedure. However, a radical prostatectomy would have a 90 day global period, and therefore all pre-operative and post-operative work for 90 days after surgery related to the prostatectomy is included in the reimbursement for the CPT code for the surgery and may not be billed separately. An E/M visit that occurs within the 90 day global that is used to address a urological problem separate from the prostatectomy may be billed when noted with the proper modifier. The global period for any particular CPT code may be found through the website for the Center for Medicare and Medicaid Services.

Modifiers

A modifier is a series of numbers or letters attached either to and E/M level of service or a CPT code to allow a provider to indicate that there is some alteration in the specific circumstances related to the code, but without changing the essential nature of the service provided by that code. This improves accurate communication of the specifics of the actual care delivered and the timing of the delivery of the care. It may improve reimbursement for services provided or prevent denial of payment for services that were in fact appropriately documented and delivered. For example, a commonly used modifier that is applied to E/M services is the 25 modifier. This allows a provider to bill for a separately identifiable E/M service that is provided on the same day as a procedure. Billing for an E/M service provided on the same day the decision to perform a surgery with a 90-day global can be accomplished by adding modifier 57 to the E/M level of service. Modifiers applied to CPT codes are more numerous and more often utilized to improve the accuracy of the surgical intervention. For example, there are modifiers that notify that a procedure was performed in a bilateral manner or on two separate structures on the same side of the body (ureteroscopy and laser lithotripsy on calculi in both the ureter and kidney would be such a case). Modifiers can help to unbundle a separately billable code when appropriate or identify when a procedure is done in a staged manner or is an unplanned procedure completed within the 90-day global for the original surgery. Modifier 51 notifies payers that multiple procedures were done during the same operative session by the same physician. If are particular case is requires increased work time or procedural complexity, then modifier 22 may be added to the CPT code to request increased reimbursement for the increased procedural service. Modifier 52 notes reduced services and may be utilized when a procedure is started but not completed, for example. Obviously, knowledge and proper employment of modifiers is critical to seeking proper reimbursement given all the complexity and nuances to the work done by a practicing urologist.

ICD-10 Codes

All the care provided by a urologist must have a reason that the service was rendered, and the ICD-10 code is the language that allows the most accurate description of the diagnosis or symptom being treated. These codes are found in the International Statistical Classification of Diseases and Related Health Problems 10th Revision. This is provided by the World Health Organization and is published yearly. Every E/M visit and each CPT code must have an associated ICD-10 code to identify the reason for the encounter or surgery. These codes allow for very detailed specificity, and accurate coding and billing depends on using the most appropriate code for the service. If a definite diagnosis is not determined yet at the time of service, one should associate symptoms instead.

Just as a medical student may initially be overwhelmed with the plethora of new terms for anatomy, physiology, and pharmacology when entering the field of medicine, the language of billing and coding may be similarly confusing and foreign to a urologist just entering practice. However, with repetition and proper continuing education to stay up to date, the provider may become just as adept this necessary aspect of medical care as providing surgery and medications.

Coding Resources

The exact manner in which a urologist goes about the daily task of coding and billing for his work will vary greatly depending on the nature of the practice setting in which he/she performs such work. In a large, multi-specialty group practice, a team of coders may be employed by the practice to perform essentially all the tasks of coding and billing, and the physician's role may be relatively limited beyond providing the actual medical care and documenting it accurately. In a single-specialty private practice setting, the urologist may be determining the level of E/M service for every patient seen and providing the CPT code for every surgery performed. Other settings may have a combination of provider input to coding with oversight and auditing by coding specialists. In each case, however, I believe it is critical for a urologist to have a good working knowledge of this topic to make sure he/she is being properly paid for the work being done, minimize the risk of fraud occurring in his/her name, and being able to have an informed and productive discussion with coders and payers when disagreements arise.

Coding Staff

If one is going to rely on others to do the work of coding and billing, then it is imperative that they have the appropriate expertise to do it effectively. A medical coder must have some understanding of anatomy and physiology as well as medical procedures in order to be able to accurately assess office visit notes and surgical reports. They must be knowledgeable in the most recent changes to the coding landscape and have the ethical foundation to identify any potentially fraudulent acts. The American Academy of Professional Coders (AAPC) provides education and certification of professional coders. Hiring coders designated as certified professional coders through this organization may help to ensure the proper level of skill and commitment necessary for optimal practice.

Working with the coding staff to identify a compliance plan, perform routine audits to quickly identify any coding or documentation errors, correct billing errors when found, and have a clear channel of communication between patients, payers, physicians and the coders are all essential elements to have a functioning urology practice. Investing in continuing education for the coders through attendance at seminars and conferences is a critical way to optimize their skills and knowledge. This should be done yearly as many new codes and rule changes are implanted on a yearly basis. Providing access to the most up to date manuals and online resources also helps the coders to do their job most effectively.

Physician Resources

The practicing urologist can acquire the skills and knowledge necessary to be an effective coding resource in a number of ways. Books and manuals, online resources, and conference attendance all play a vital role in maintaining effectiveness in the business of medicine. A physician must apply the same level of interest to this aspect of the practice as he/she does to journal reading and conference attendance to continue providing excellent and contemporary medical care to the patient population.

Reference manuals that should be obtained yearly include the latest CPT book, ICD-10 manual, Healthcare Common Procedure Coding System for being able to report services for supplies and drugs, and National Correct Coding Initiative to stay up to date on bundling edits. The wall chart and pocket card to determine appropriate E/M level determination should be readily available as a reference.

The American Urological Association (AUA) provides several services to urology practices that are an invaluable resource for handling difficult coding challenges and maintaining proper knowledge of this topic. The AUA Coding Hotline allows an online or telephone interaction for access to professional coders at the AUA to help with particularly challenging coding situations [4, 5]. The AUA Coding Today is an online subscription product developed by Physician Reimbursement Systems and co-sponsored by the AUA. This service provides CPT and ICD-10 codes, current bundling edits, information on global days and modifier usage, AUA coding tips, and even local coverage decisions. The AUA holds an annual coding seminar that provides an intensive education in the basics of coding as well as critical updates that can affect a urology practice. It is designed to benefit both coders and physicians. I believe it is critical for every urologist to attend this early in his/her career to gain an appreciation for the complexity and depth of this topic. While a young physician may be overwhelmed and confused at the first attendance of this meeting, yearly attendance reinforces critical elements to the coding and billing process and allows the development of expertise to be brought back to the practice.

Coding and billing talks are also part of many urological continuing education conferences and should be attended with the same enthusiasm and attention as talks on urological oncology or other conditions. I have found presentations by Dr. Ray Painter and Dr. Michael Ferragamo to be particularly helpful and accessible for a novice in coding and billing. The PRS Network also presents coding seminars for a fee that provide yet another in person resource for additional education [6–10].

While proper coding and billing may be given little attention in urology graduate medical education, it is critical to the success of any urological practice. A solid grasp of the fundamentals of this topic combined with a commitment to purse ongoing education should allow a urologist to obtain proper reimbursement for work done and minimize the risk of committing fraud and abuse.

References

1. Painter, R, Proper Billing and Coding, in D. Kursh, Elroy & C. Ulchaker, James. (2001). Office Urology: The Clinician's Guide. https://doi.org/10.1007/978-1-59259-010-0.
2. Stinchcomb SN, Coding and reimbursement: the lifeline of the urologist's office. Urol Clin North Am. 2005;32(3):285–90, vi.
3. Dowling RA, Painter M. Coding for urologic office procedures. Urol Clin North Am. 2013;40 (4):599–611. https://doi.org/10.1016/j.ucl.2013.07.011 Epub 2013 Sep 11.
4. www.auanet.org.
5. www.auacodingtoday.com.
6. www.prsnetwork.com.
7. www.rvsdata.com.
8. www.cms.gov.
9. www.ama-assn.org.
10. www.aapc.com.

Chapter 14
Telemedicine in Urology

Gregory W. Hosier and Thomas Chi

Introduction

Medicine has been undergoing a digital transformation and telemedicine is one important dimension of this transformation that urologists need to understand and embrace. Just as the music industry saw the onset of digital music transition from in-person retail stores to online streaming platforms, telemedicine also allows the patient–physician encounter to proceed in a virtual and remote environment. The music industry also serves as a stark reminder. Leading into the twenty-first century, HMV (for "His Master's Voice," originally a British music and entertainment retailer) was one of the largest global music retailers. By 2013, HMV would file for bankruptcy after nearly 100 years in business. Spotify was started in 2006 and provided a convenient, online platform to access a vast digital music catalog allowing music consumers to enjoy their purchases from the convenience of their home or location of choice. Contrary to the fate of HMV, Spotify in 2021 reported over 365 million monthly active users from 178 different countries [1]. In the field of medicine, over the past decade, advances in technology have facilitated the expansion of telemedicine. These were accelerated in 2020 with the onset of the COVID-19 pandemic response where the use of telemedicine expanded greatly as it offered a safe and convenient way to provide ongoing care to patients. Similar to digital music streaming services, now that the convenience of telemedicine for both patients and providers has been realized, it must be understood and embraced by the practicing urologist to better serve our patients and our communities.

G. W. Hosier · T. Chi (✉)
University of California San Francisco Department of Urology, 400 Parnassus Avenue A610, San Francisco, CA 94143, USA
e-mail: tom.chi@ucsf.edu

Definitions

Although often used interchangeably, the terms telehealth, telemedicine, and virtual care all have different definitions [3, 4]. Telehealth is the broadest term and refers to the use of virtual platforms to facilitate patient care, education, monitoring, and prevention [4]. Telemedicine more specifically refers to the use of technology to interface directly with providers and patients. Virtual care refers to any interaction between providers and patients using virtual technology to improve the quality and effectiveness of patient care [4]. Examples of virtual care include messaging between patient and provider, remote monitoring of patients, and communication between members of the health care team to provide continuity and accessibility of care [4].

Further distinctions are made whether the interaction occurs in real time (synchronous) such as phone/video-conferencing, or if data is recorded and transmitted for later interpretation (asynchronous) [3, 4]. Some literature also makes a distinction between physician–physician interactions (e.g., tumor boards) and direct-to-consumer interactions (e.g., telemedicine visits, patient phone calls) [3]. Urologic clinical practice is well positioned to take advantage of all of these various types of telehealth mechanisms to enhance patient care.

Regulation, Reimbursement, and Technology

Regulation

Telemedicine regulations vary state-to-state. Rules differ regarding the establishment of a valid doctor–patient relationship, consent requirements, and whether a provider must be in physical proximity to the patient. Prior to 2017, state licensure required that a patient be treated in the state where the patient resides. During that time period, telemedicine could only be delivered between providers and patients within state lines. This was streamlined somewhat by 29 states participating in the Interstate Medical Licensure Compact of 2017, but these interstate restrictions were a factor that contributed to poor adoption rates of telemedicine within most medical communities. In 2020, motivated by the COVID-19 pandemic onset, most states adopted temporary mechanisms to allow out-of-state physicians to rapidly acquire licensure. These regulatory changes coupled with a shift toward improved reimbursement for telemedicine encounters drove significantly increased uptake of telemedicine not only within urology, but across medical fields. In 2022, states have shifted toward re-establishing interstate licensure restrictions which may impact practitioners' ability to provide telemedicine care across state lines. It is unclear to what capacity, if at all, these regulatory changes will persist in the future. To fully leverage telemedicine within one's clinical practice, it is important to familiarize oneself with state-specific guidelines and updates. Providers are encouraged to seek guidance from their state medical board regarding telemedicine regulation.

Reimbursement

Leading up to 2020, Medicare and private payers were increasingly covering telemedicine services and relaxing restrictions on the use of telemedicine. Parallel to the significant relaxation of interstate licensure regulation that occurred during the public health emergency period beginning in 2020, most major private payers began providing telemedicine reimbursement across the entire nation. In March 2020, the Centers for Medicare and Medicaid Services introduced waiver 1135, which radically expanded reimbursement for telemedical services [5].

Within the 1135 waiver, there is a distinction made between telehealth visits, virtual check-ins, e-visits, and e-consults [5]. Table 14.1. provides a brief explanation of each. Telehealth visits refer to synchronous visits between provider and patient. These can be between new or established patients. Virtual check-ins are short 5–10 min communications intended only for patients with an established relationship with their provider. These can be synchronous or asynchronous and are often initiated by the patient. Examples include phone call, teleconferencing, secure text messaging, or secure email. For billing purposes, these cannot be related to a visit within the previous 7 days or lead to an appointment within 24 h. E-visits are restricted to established patients, must be initiated by patients, and involve communications between provider and patient using an online portal. For billing purposes, a provider response must occur within 7 days. E-consults refer to written electronic communications between a referring provider and consulting physician involving a review of a patient's medical record and treatment recommendations. All of these telehealth mechanisms can be deployed in clinical practice to maximize patient access to care while still representing avenues by which clinical work can be reimbursed. This paradigm shift is important to understand and embrace. Many of these activities previously occupied non-billable clinician time and were, therefore, underutilized. Incorporating them fully into urologic practice can increase patient care access.

Technology

The United States federal government also changed, in 2020, the restrictions on the technology platforms that can be used for telemedicine. Providers have always been encouraged to use platforms that are compliant with the Health Insurance Portability and Accountability Act (HIPAA) of 1996, such as Doxy.me and Zoom for Healthcare. However, to improve patient access when COVID-19 pandemic

Table 14.1 Current procedural terminology (CPT) and Healthcare Common Procedure Coding System (HCPCS) codes for telehealth, virtual check-ins, e-visits, and e-consults

Codes	Descriptor	New Patient	Established Patient
Telehealth			
99,201–99,215	Office or other outpatient visits	X	X
G0425-G0427	Telehealth consultations, emergency department or initial inpatient	X	X
G0406-408	Follow-up, or inpatient consultation via Telehealth		X
Virtual Check-In			
G2010	Remote evaluation of recorded video and/or images (e.g., store and forward), including interpretation with follow-up with the patient within 24 business hours, not originating from a related service provided within the previous 7 days nor leading to a service within the next 24 h; 5–10 min		X
G2012	Brief communication technology-based service by a physician or other qualified health care professional who can report evaluation and management services, not originating from a related service provided within the previous 7 days nor leading to a service within the next 24 h or soonest available appointment; 5–10 min		X
E-Visits			
99421–99423	Online digital evaluation and management service for up to 7 days		X
G2061–G2063	Online assessment by qualified non-physician healthcare professional		X
E-Consults			
99446–99452	Interprofessional telephone/Internet/electronic health assessment and management service provided by a consultative physician, including a verbal and written report to the patient's treating/requesting physician or other qualified health care professional; 5–10 min	X	X

pressures increased the need for telehealth accessibility, the Office for Civil Rights liberalized its enforcement of the Portability and Accountability Act of 1996 through the provision of telemedicine services. Providers became permitted to use any non-public facing platform that allows the sharing of information without access to the general public. Table 14.2. provides examples of non-public facing platforms. This is in contrast to public facing platforms in which communications are viewable to the general public, such as Instagram and Facebook.

Table 14.2 Examples of non-public facing video and text services used for telemedicine

Video	Text	HIPPA Compliant
Zoom for Healthcare	TigerText	Yes
Doxy.me	Zinc	Yes
GoToMeeting	Spok Mobile	Yes
SimplePractice Telehealth	OhMD	Yes
VSee	VSee	Yes
SecureVideo	Rocket.chat	Yes
Microsoft Teams	Microsoft Teams	Can be configured
Cisco Jabber	Cisco Jabber	Can be configured
Apple FaceTime	iMessage	No
Facebook Messenger	Facebook Messenger	No
WhatsApp video	WhatsApp	No
Skype		No
Google Hangouts		No

HIPPA, Health Insurance Portability and Accountability Act

Telemedicine Use in Urology

A 2016 American Medical Association survey found that pathology, emergency medicine, and psychiatry utilized telemedicine the most, while urology was among the specialties that utilized telemedicine the least [6]. In 2020, the emergence of the COVID-19 pandemic greatly expanded the use of telemedicine within all fields of medicine, including urology, to facilitate social distancing, continue patient care, and support financial viability for practices. In the 2020 AUA census, 71.5% of urologists stated that they participated in telemedicine during the pandemic. The most common telemedicine encounter diagnoses were benign prostatic hyperplasia, elevated prostate-specific antigen, erectile dysfunction, stone disease, and voiding dysfunction. Approximately half of the urologists provided telemedicine encounters for new patients and 77% provided encounters for established patients. Of those urologists who utilized telemedicine, compensation was primarily for video visits (93.9%) and telephone calls (77%), whereas fewer than 11% reported receiving compensation for e-consults, video visits with other providers, or text messages [7]. These survey data demonstrate that urologists have been able to apply telemedicine to a wide variety of patients within clinical practice.

Evidence for Telemedicine in Urology

Even before the emergence of the COVID-19 pandemic in 2020, there were a number of studies evaluating the use of telemedicine in urology. A systematic review by Edison et al. found two randomized controlled trials, 10 prospective studies, and six retrospective studies, spanning the majority of urologic sub-specialties including uro-oncology, endourology, general urology, and functional urology. These studies consistently showed high rates of patient satisfaction, with no increase in complications, and a referral rate for in-person visits of approximately one-in-three, indicating that roughly two-thirds of cases can be completely managed through telemedicine [8].

In one of the first randomized controlled trials of telemedicine in urology, Viers et al. compared virtual visits to in-person visits in 70 patients after radical prostatectomy and found no difference in total time spent on care (mean 17.9 vs. 17.8 min, 95% CI 5.9–5.6; $P = 0.97$), total clinician–patient contact time (12.1 vs. 11.8 min, 95% CI 4.2–3.5; $P = 0.85$), patient wait-time (18.4 vs. 13.0 min, 95% CI 13.7–3.0; $P = 0.20$), patient satisfaction (88% vs. 91%, $P = 0.7$), or clinician satisfaction (88% vs. 90%) [9]. While one limitation of this study was the possible risk of selection bias given that only 24% of screened patients were enrolled, these results overall highlight that urology as a specialty is well positioned for telehealth implementation.

These shifts in the medical landscape have led to a significant increase in telemedicine utilization. Subsequently, many benefits and some barriers to implementing telemedicine have been identified.

Benefits of Telemedicine

Benefits of telemedicine include increased efficiency for providers and patients. An important efficiency metric used to evaluate business practices is cycle time. When applied to medicine, cycle time comprises patient check-in, time spent waiting before seeing a provider, patient–physician interaction, and checkout. For video visits, these elements are simplified and include signing in to the visit, interacting with a urologist, and logging off. In one Michigan study of 250 telemedicine visits and 250 in-person visits, cycle time for video visits was 24 min compared to 80-min for in-person visits ($p < 0.01$) [5]. There is evidence that increased convenience for patients translates into improved follow-up compliance. Shanbehzadeh et al. found that patients were more compliant with 3 to 5 month telemedicine follow-ups compared to in-person follow-ups (90.1% vs. 79.3%, p = 0.04) [10].

Additional benefits for patients include decreased time and travel costs. In one study from the Veterans Affairs Greater Los Angeles Healthcare System, patients saved an average of 277 travel miles, 290 min of travel time, $67 in travel expenses, and $126 in lost opportunity cost when utilizing telehealth as opposed to in-person visits [11]. Taken together, these data demonstrate that telemedicine patients experience highly satisfactory visits associated with a decreased personal cost for them. When efficient care can be delivered at low cost and high levels of patient satisfaction, value can be achieved.

This value can also be considered for its impact on care systems. Decreased travel has the added benefit of lowering the annual carbon footprint. Conversion to telemedicine visits has been shown to result in a decrease of 0.7 to 4.35 metric tons of CO_2 emissions [11, 12]. In addition, telemedicine should intuitively decrease the cost of the system by forgoing costs related to clinic space, staffing, and resources. Some have raised concerns that these savings may be limited by two mechanisms that should be considered by all urologists. Firstly, some telemedicine visits may require an additional in-person visit resulting in two visits instead of one. Secondly, the convenience of telemedicine may lead to increased utilization by patients leading to increased costs. To increase understanding of these two issues, Nord et al. conducted a survey immediately following telehealth visits, asking patients what care they would have sought if telehealth had not been an option [13]. The team then conducted a follow-up survey 1–2 weeks after each patient's visit to see if any follow-up care had been pursued. The survey found that 16% would have "done nothing" if the telehealth visit had not been an option and that 75% did not seek any follow-up care. After accounting for increased utilization and follow-up care, the overall net cost savings was $19–121, with the most cost savings coming from avoiding emergency department visits [13]. As can be seen, telemedicine value can also be derived for the environment as well as the cost of the health care system.

Of particular interest for urologists, whose practice can entail a large number of procedures performed in the clinic, shifting clinical visits to a telemedicine format can free up resources to allow quicker access and increased capacity for in-person procedures. To demonstrate this concept, we integrated telehealth into clinic schedules by shifting the bulk of our clinic visits for new and existing patients to be conducted via televideo in the spring of 2020. This allowed in-person visits to focus on primary procedures, reimaging the clinic as a purely procedure-oriented space, akin to an outpatient surgery center. This change facilitated a COVID-19 pandemic response allowing for socially distanced clinical care in the clinic, and the impact of this change was measured. In a 5 months period prior to this reimagining of the clinic, 93% of patient visits were conducted in person, of which 8% were for procedures. In 5 months period after the change was made, 50% of total visits were seen in person, of which 45% were for procedures. This resulted in 70% of new patients being scheduled within 14 days compared to 46% prior to this change. It also corresponded with a slight improvement in patient satisfaction (unpublished) highlighting the idea that effective incorporation of telemedicine can increase urologists' ability to provide procedures to patients at a higher volume in an ambulatory clinic setting.

Barriers to Telemedicine

In a systematic review, the most commonly reported barriers to implementing telemedicine were concerns with reimbursement and poor technological literacy of providers [14]. With the increasing utilization of telemedicine, these barriers are being overcome.

Although urologists are by and large more comfortable with the use of telemedicine, barriers still remain to ongoing use through technology disruptions and workflow inefficiencies. Cohen et al. observed 23 telemedicine video visits and quantified disruptions or system inefficiencies during these visits [15]. The most common barriers to effective use were interruptions (15%), communication breakdown (15%), and poor internet connectivity (14%) [15]. As providers and patients become more familiar with telemedicine platforms, it is expected that these disruptions and inefficiencies will further improve.

One major barrier for both providers and patients as telemedicine users is the lack of access to broadband internet and smart devices. This can affect people living in rural and urban settings alike. For example, up to 48% of households in Bronx neighborhoods do not have broadband internet access [16]. When considering patient access, disparities in Internet access worsen when stratifying the population by race, age, and poverty level. Along these three axes, studies have shown that 30% of Hispanic and Black vs 20% of White and Asian patients, 42% of seniors older than 65 years versus 23% of patients ages 18 to 24 years, and 44% of people living below the poverty level for income versus 22% above report no access to adequate internet or devices to permit telemedicine utilization [16–18]. This raises ethical concerns about the unequal distribution of health care resources, which could further widen racial and socioeconomic disparities in care.

While these disparities issues can be challenging to address, tools exist for the practicing urologist to consider. One option to help alleviate these disparities includes engaging family members and friends to assist during the telehealth appointment. Within a patient's social network, pooled resources may find access to necessary technology for telemedicine encounters. Studies have also shown that most patients who do not have the technological capability to participate in video visits can still participate in telephone visits [18]. Another option is to utilize primary-care offices with appropriate broadband access to enable patients to access specialty care through telehealth. The first step toward advancing access to care despite adversity is to recognize and address challenges creatively and collaboratively.

Urologic Conditions Best Suited for Telemedicine

When considering whether a consultation is appropriate to see via telemedicine, it is useful to ask oneself three questions. First, will physical exam findings alone meaningfully alter the management course for this patient? Second, will this consultation require a procedure to be performed? Third, is bad news being delivered that may benefit from a comforting in-person presence? If answers to each of these questions are no, then the consultation is generally well suited to telemedicine.

In a prospective, multisite study of 1679 telehealth appointments, 18 adult and pediatric urologists covering all urologic sub-specialties were asked whether appointments resulted in complete, suboptimal, or incomplete (requiring in-person visit) case management [19]. Endourology cases had the highest rate of complete case management (86%), while cases with a firm diagnosis of cancer, and adult functional/andrology urology cases had moderately high complete case management rates (72–73%) [19]. Cases in which cancer was suspected but not yet diagnosed (53%) and pediatric cases (38%) had the lowest rates of complete case management [19]. Encouragingly, two-thirds of cases were felt to be completely managed virtually and only 2–6% were felt to require an in-person visit [19]. Similarly, Luciano et al., found that the majority of patients with cancer suspicion still required in-person visits. Patient satisfaction was reportedly not different among general urology, andrology, endourology, and oncology cases [20].

Although authors did not examine conditions within pediatric urology that were felt to be better suited to telemedicine, other studies have shown that neonatal, voiding dysfunction, reflux, infections, and post-operative visits are well suited, while conditions such as undescended testes in which a physical exam is important are less well suited to telemedicine [21]. Interestingly, patient/parent satisfaction remains very high for pediatric telemedicine visits even if providers feel the case management was suboptimal, likely due to minimization of time/travel/cost barriers to parents which can be significant for in-person visits [19, 21]. Figure 14.1 presents a framework for what conditions and patient encounter types might lend themselves to telemedicine or not. When thinking of ways to incorporate telehealth into one's practice, urologists should consider multiple dimensions that take into account both provider and patient needs.

Incorporating Physician Extenders into Telemedicine Visits

An additional challenge for many urologists who work with either advanced practice providers (APPs) or trainees has been how best to incorporate these physician extenders into a telemedicine clinic flow. In 2020, a number of guidance documents were established to aid with this [22]. The most commonly recommended approach, and one we have found effective at our institution, is to follow a similar workflow to in-person encounters (Fig. 14.2) [23]. The APP or trainee can

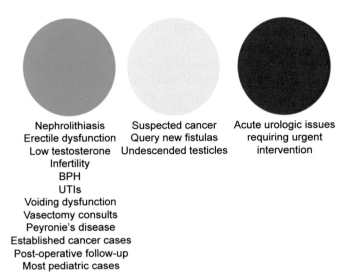

Nephrolithiasis	Suspected cancer	Acute urologic issues
Erectile dysfunction	Query new fistulas	requiring urgent
Low testosterone	Undescended testicles	intervention

Infertility
BPH
UTIs
Voiding dysfunction
Vasectomy consults
Peyronie's disease
Established cancer cases
Post-operative follow-up
Most pediatric cases

Fig. 14.1 Conditions that lend themselves well to telemedicine visits (green), conditions that may benefit from in-person consultation (yellow), and conditions in which telemedicine visits are generally not recommended (red)

first interview the patient and then present the case to the supervising urologist. This can be accomplished using a variety of technology platforms that allow the patient or the physician extender to be moved between virtual spaces. After cases have been discussed, both supervising urologist and physician extender can then see the patient together and complete the visit. In the virtual environment, documentation requirements and workflows in the context of working with physician extenders remain largely unchanged. Choosing a technology platform that allows for virtual waiting rooms and breakout rooms allows many different options to incorporate physician extenders into synchronous patient care. These can be adapted to fit many urologists' workflows.

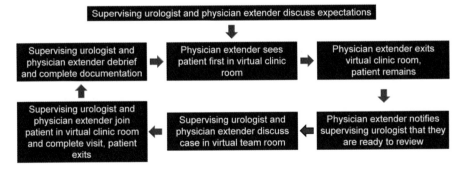

Fig. 14.2 An example of a telemedicine clinic workflow for supervising urologist and physician extender

Telementoring and Telesurgery

Exciting dimensions that telehealth has introduced into clinical practice include telementoring and telesurgery. With telehealth driving advances in telecommunications technologies, simultaneous growth in robotic surgery has greatly facilitated advancement in these areas. Telementoring refers to an expert watching a real-time video feed of an operation being performed by another surgeon in a different geographic location and providing guidance. Telesurgery refers to a surgeon operating on a patient from a remote site.

In a proof of concept study for telementoring, Hinata and colleagues showed no difference in operating time, complication rate, early continence status, and positive margin rate among two surgeons who underwent telementoring compared to two surgeons who underwent in-person mentoring for 30 initial robotic-assisted laparoscopic radical prostatectomy (RALP) cases. All four surgeons had experience with open radical prostatectomy and had undergone robotic training provided by the manufacturer, but had not previously performed RALP [24]. Telementoring offers a substantial benefit for learners of all levels by reducing travel time and cost for mentors and could revolutionize the way surgeons are licensed and credentialed to practice urology.

The first published example of telesurgery was a transrectal ultrasound guided prostate biopsy performed by Rovetta and Sala in 1995 [25]. The first complete telesurgical operation, known as the "Lindbergh operation", was a robotic cholecystectomy performed by a group of French surgeons in New York on a patient located in Strasbourg, France [26]. In urology, the use of telesurgery was reported for robotic percutaneous renal puncture for stone treatment in 2001 [27]. Overall, reports of telesurgery have been mostly limited to use in animals, but with time we will likely see applications in clinical practice [25]. One area where telesurgery implementation may be extremely useful is in remote locations without access to specialized surgical services.

Achieving this future state of telesurgery will require addressing multiple barriers. Among them include safety, legal, and billings concerns. Safety concerns include latency time between the origin and remote sites as well as the possibility of technology failure and the need to convert to an open approach. Bove et al., reported in 2003 that, in 5 of 17 planned telementoring/telesurgery procedures, a connection to the remote site could not be established [28]. In two of 17 cases, conversion to open procedure was required [28]. With advances in telecommunication including widespread expansion of 5G capabilities, connection issues are anticipated to be less of an issue. However, the potential need for open conversion remains a concern. An additional safety concern is a possibility of a cyberattack. In an analysis of the Raven II surgical platform, authors found that the system was vulnerable to attacks that could result in manipulation of the surgical arms, or delay of transmission of the surgeon's actions to the surgical arms [29]. Billing and licensure concerns also exist when working across state and national borders, which remain a barrier for telesurgery. Nevertheless, with the field of urology facing an aging workforce and future shortages, telementoring and telesurgery will be exciting areas to support increased access to care that move telehealth toward the future of medicine.

The Future of Telemedicine in Urology

Similar to how streaming services transformed the landscape of music retail, telemedicine is rapidly shifting the care paradigm for the practicing urologist. According to the 2018 AUA census data, 30% of urologists are greater than 65 years old, making urology the second oldest surgical specialty behind thoracic surgery [18]. By 2030, it is anticipated that urology will face a 32% shortage (18). Telemedicine can be a patient satisfier that will offer value to clinical practice and may help alleviate an anticipated urology workforce shortage by allowing access to care for patients who otherwise do not have a local urologist. Implementing equal access to telemedical services remains an important area for future progress. Embracing telemedicine will allow the contemporary urologist to move toward the future of urological practice.

Key Points

- Use of telemedicine within urology has greatly expanded over time. While remuneration and regulation policies have been relaxed to support wider adoption, urologists should remain abreast of updates in these areas.
- Telemedicine offers benefits including decreased time and travel costs for patients, increased follow-up compliance, and potential cost savings for the healthcare system.
- Disparities in access to telemedical services exist. Identifying methods to decrease gaps in access remains an important area for consideration.
- Most urologic conditions are well suited to telemedicine visits. Exceptions include cases in which the physical exam may greatly impact management (such as undescended testicles), cases involving breaking bad news (such as new/ suspected cancer diagnoses), or conditions that may require urgent intervention (such as urinary retention or acute scrotum).
- Physician extenders can be successfully integrated into telemedicine visits using a similar workflow to traditional in-person encounters (physician extender sees patient and presents the case to the supervising urologist, then both can see the patient and complete the visit).
- Telementoring and telesurgery are currently being explored to provide improved access to surgical training and surgical services, and may represent future keystones of clinical training and practice.
- Telemedicine may help alleviate a future anticipated shortage of urologists in the United States.

References

1. Spotify. Company info. For the Record. 2021.
2. Ovide S. Streaming saved music. Artists hate it. New York Times. 2021.
3. Ellimoottil C, Andino JJ, Mukundi S. Telemedicine in urology AUA Updat Ser. 2018;37:272–8.
4. Mechanic OJ, Persaud Y, Kimball AB. Telehealth Systems. StatPearls [Internet]. 2020 Sep 18 [cited 2021 Sep 9]; Available from: https://www.ncbi.nlm.nih.gov/books/NBK459384/.
5. Medicare telemedicine health care provider fact sheet. Centers for Medicare and Mediaide Services. [Internet]. 2020. Available from: https://www.cms.gov/newsroom/fact-sheets/medicare-telemedicine-health-care-provider-fact-sheet.
6. Kane C, Gillis K. The Use Of Telemedicine By Physicians: Still The Exception Rather Than The Rule. Health Aff (Millwood) [Internet]. 2018 Dec 1 [cited 2021 Sep 8];37(12):1923–30. Available from: https://pubmed.ncbi.nlm.nih.gov/30633670/.
7. Gettman M, Kirshenbaum E, Rhee E, Spitz A. Telemedicine in Urology. AUA White Pap. 2021.
8. Edison MA, Connor MJ, Miah S, THusseiny El, Winkler M, Dasgupta R, et al. Understanding virtual urology clinics: a systematic review. BJU Int. 2020;126(5):536–46.
9. Viers BR, Lightner DJ, Rivera ME, Tollefson MK, Boorjian SA, Karnes RJ, et al. Efficiency, satisfaction, and costs for remote video visits following radical prostatectomy: A randomized controlled trial. Eur Urol [Internet]. 2015;68(4):729–35. Available from: http://dx.doi.org/https://doi.org/10.1016/j.eururo.2015.04.002.
10. Giusto L, Derisavifard S, Zahner P, Rueb J, Deyi L, Jiayi L, et al. Telemedicine follow-up is safe and efficacious for synthetic midurethral slings: a randomized, multi-institutional control trial. Int Urogynecol J [Internet]. 2021 [cited 2021 Sep 8]; Available from: https://pubmed.ncbi.nlm.nih.gov/33877376/.
11. Chu S, Boxer R, Madison P, Kleinman L, Skolarus T, Altman L, et al. Veterans Affairs Telemedicine: Bringing Urologic Care to Remote Clinics. Urology [Internet]. 2015 Aug 1 [cited 2021 Sep 16];86(2):255–61. Available from: https://pubmed.ncbi.nlm.nih.gov/26168998/.
12. Connor M, Miah S, Edison M, Brittain J, Smith M, Hanna M, et al. Clinical, fiscal and environmental benefits of a specialist-led virtual ureteric colic clinic: a prospective study. BJU Int [Internet]. 2019 Dec 1 [cited 2021 Sep 17];124(6):1034–9. Available from: https://pubmed.ncbi.nlm.nih.gov/31206221/.
13. Nord G, Rising K, Band R, Carr B, Hollander J. On-demand synchronous audio video telemedicine visits are cost effective. Am J Emerg Med [Internet]. 2019 May 1 [cited 2021 Sep 17];37(5):890–4. Available from: https://pubmed.ncbi.nlm.nih.gov/30100333/.
14. Castaneda P, Ellimoottil C. Current use of telehealth in urology: a review. World J Urol [Internet]. 2020 Oct 1 [cited 2021 Sep 8];38(10):2377–84. Available from: https://pubmed.ncbi.nlm.nih.gov/31352565/.
15. Cohen TN, Choi E, Kanji FF, Scott VCS, Eilber KS, Anger JT. Patient and Provider Experience with Telemedicine in a Urology Practice: Identifying Opportunities for Improvement. Urol Pract. 2021;8(3):328–36.
16. New York City Comptroller: Census and the City:Overcoming NTC's Digital Divide in the 2020 Census. https://comptroller.nyc.gov/reports/census-and-the-city/. 2019.
17. Marra G, Gomez F, Cussenot O. "Virtually Perfect" for Some but Perhaps Not for All: Launching Telemedicine in the Bronx during the COVID-19 Pandemic. Letter J Urol. 2021;206(1):176–7.
18. Kirshenbaum E, Rhee EY, Gettman M, Spitz A. Telemedicine in Urology: The Socioeconomic Impact. Urol Clin North Am [Internet]. 2021;48(2):215–22. Available from: https://doi.org/10.1016/j.ucl.2021.01.006.

19. Turcotte B, Paquet S, Blais AS, Blouin AC, Bolduc S, Bureau M, et al. A prospective, multisite study analyzing the percentage of urological cases that can be completely managed by telemedicine. Can Urol Assoc J. 2020;14(10):319–21.
20. Shiff B, Frankel J, Oake J, Blachman-Braun R, Patel P. Patient Satisfaction With Telemedicine Appointments in an Academic Andrology-focused Urology Practice During the COVID-19 Pandemic. Urology [Internet]. 2021;153:35–41. Available from: https://doi.org/10.1016/j.urology.2020.11.065.
21. Winkelman AJ, Beller HL, Morgan KE, Corbett ST, Leroy S V., Noona SW, et al. Benefits and barriers to pediatric tele-urology during the COVID-19 pandemic. J Pediatr Urol [Internet]. 2020 Dec 1 [cited 2021 Sep 15];16(6):840.e1. Available from: /pmc/articles/PMC7543732/.
22. Canadian Medical Association. Virtual Care Playbook. 2020.
23. Iancu AM, Kemp MT, Gribbin W, Liesman DR, Nevarez J, Pinsky A, et al. Twelve tips for the integration of medical students into telemedicine visits. Med Teach [Internet]. 2020;0(0):1–7. Available from: https://doi.org/10.1080/0142159X.2020.1844877.
24. Hinata N, Miyake H, Kurahashi T, Ando M, Furukawa J, Ishimura T, et al. Novel Telementoring System for Robot-assisted Radical Prostatectomy: Impact on the Learning Curve. Urology. 2014 May 1;83(5):1088–92.
25. Hung AJ, Chen J, Shah A, Gill IS. Telementoring and Telesurgery for Minimally Invasive Procedures. J Urol [Internet]. 2018;199(2):355–69. Available from: https://doi.org/10.1016/j.juro.2017.06.082.
26. Marescaux J, Leroy J, Gagner M, Rubino F, Mutter D, Vix M, et al. Transatlantic robot-assisted telesurgery. Nature [Internet]. 2001 Sep 27 [cited 2021 Sep 24];413(6854):379–80. Available from: https://pubmed.ncbi.nlm.nih.gov/11574874/.
27. Bauer J, Lee B, Stoianovici D, Bishoff J, Micali S, Micali L, et al. Remote percutaneous renal access using a new automated telesurgical robotic system. Telemed J E Health [Internet]. 2001 [cited 2021 Sep 24];7(4):341–6. Available from: https://pubmed.ncbi.nlm.nih.gov/11886670/.
28. Bove P, Stoianovici D, Micali S, Patriciu A, Grassi N, Jarrett TW, et al. Is telesurgery a new reality? Our experience with laparoscopic and percutaneous procedures. J Endourol. 2003;17(3):137–42.
29. Bonaci T, Herron J, Yusuf T, Yan J, Kohno T, Chizeck HJ. To Make a Robot Secure: An Experimental Analysis of Cyber Security Threats Against Teleoperated Surgical Robots. 2015;1–11. Available from: http://arxiv.org/abs/1504.04339.

Chapter 15
Time Management

Woodson W. Smelser, Aaron A. Laviana, and Sam S. Chang

Introduction

"He who knows most grieves most for wasted time".

—Dante [1].

It is almost impossible to encounter someone who does not feel at some point that he or she has too much to handle and/or not enough time to get it all done. From the provider tasked with making dozens of calls and emails after the office closes while simultaneously completing electronic medical charts, completing insurance paperwork, and reviewing test results to the staff having to handle the inadequate standard appointment time of fifteen minutes to the nursing manager having to handle 100-plus email requests per day; everyone is flooded by what seems like an innumerable number of "urgent requests". Interestingly, a paradox has also developed over the new millennium. People have made attempts to enhance their quality of life but frequently add to their stress levels by taking on more than they have the time and/or resources to handle [2]. This self-imposed increase in responsibilities frustrates and antagonizes an already perplexing situation. A survey of almost 7 million people in the United States revealed that Americans reported

Senior Author: Sam S. Chang.

W. W. Smelser (✉) · S. S. Chang
Department of Urology, Vanderbilt University Medical Center, Nashville, TN, USA
e-mail: woodson.w.smelser@vumc.org

S. S. Chang
e-mail: sam.chang@vumc.org

A. A. Laviana
Department of Surgery and Perioperative Care, The University of Texas at Austin Dell Medical School, Austin, TX, USA
e-mail: aaron.laviana@austin.utexas.edu

© The Author(s), under exclusive license to Springer Nature Switzerland AG 2022
S. Y. Nakada and S. R. Patel (eds.), *Navigating Organized Urology*,
https://doi.org/10.1007/978-3-031-05540-9_15

substantially higher levels of depressive symptoms, particularly somatic symptoms, in the 2000s–2010s versus the 1980s–1990s [3]. Even more recently, the broad and intense stressors of the COVID-19 global pandemic have motivated many health-care workers to re-evaluate their overall work quality of life [4, 5]. Recent studies into the stresses associated with work roles during the pandemic have found that 40% have experienced new financial stress, 41% report loneliness and isolation, and 62% report that they are too tired to perform basic household duties when they return home from work, leading to increased strain on family members and partners [5]. Furthermore, 34% of healthcare workers reported taking out their stress on their children and partners, and 53% reported experiencing burnout [5]. Finally, of those healthcare providers with children, 32% reported not having enough time or emotional bandwidth to spend adequate time with their children [5]. The long-term effects of these findings are undetermined, but clearly from these results, taking more time for family, pursuing parallel interests, and learning new skills are all pursuits that may be prioritized in addition to a busy career as a urologist as a result of the pandemic.

Improving time management is believed to decrease stress and improve efficiency, clinical effectiveness, and patient care. As Benjamin Franklin first attested 250 years ago, "time is money" [6]. This concept is as salient as ever today, and as urologists, we must have a firm grasp on good time management skills to maximize success in all facets of life. While there is no universal solution, seminar, or app that will improve everyone's time management, there are ways to facilitate improvements in personal productivity and organization; and with this are some simple processes that everyone can use to maximize output and minimize input in a world where work is increasingly volume centric. The purpose of this chapter is to focus on methods to increase one's self-awareness of time management while discussing techniques to prioritize tasks more effectively to achieve as healthy a work-life balance as possible.

Background

The desire for improved efficiency and time management is far from novel. The earliest measurements of the time trace back to pre-sixteenth Century BC when there was a basic understanding of sunrises, sunsets, and seasonal changes [7]. The idea of time slowly reformed over the ensuing centuries with St. Benedictine Monks being the first known individuals to schedule daily activities at particular times of the day in the Sixth Century. Nevertheless, one of the most formative pendulum shifts occurred during the Industrial Revolution in the eighteenth and nineteenth centuries. John Letts produced the first commercial diary in 1812 to provide local merchants and traders with a way to track tides and record financial transactions [8]. Shortly thereafter, wristwatches and time clocks were developed, which placed even a stronger emphasis on time. These pivotal inventions eventually paved the way for the creation of the assembly line by Ransom Olds and Henry

Ford. By assigning specific roles and tracking times, the assembly line substantially increased productivity by decreasing the car assembly time from 12.5 to 1.5 man-hours. This success was a major driver in Henry Ford's decision to decrease the workday from 9 to 8 h while doubling pay from $2.25 to $5 per day [9]. Similar trends and improvements in time management were seen across industries, and eventually, the first book on this topic was written by James Mckay in 1958 [10]. Since then, countless books have been written on time management, each focusing on some element of time analysis, planning, goal setting, prioritizing, and scheduling. Implementing all of these strategies at once is not feasible, but successful adoption of one or two may prove fruitful over the long run. The remainder of this chapter focuses on techniques to improve time management, and these techniques are categorized into two major groups:

1. **Setting Priorities**.
2. **Minimizing Distractions**.

Section 1: Setting Priorities

Despite a plethora of self-help books and available material on this topic, none of these techniques will work unless a person is motivated to use them. Importantly, many people who struggle to manage their time effectively will not want to take the additional time to read advice, and as such, effective time management is as much psychological as it is incorporating tangible methods. In truth, one must stay highly motivated to maintain an organized approach to work, especially when encountering time constraints, requests, emails, calls, interruptions, and unexpected roadblocks [11].

Set compelling goals and eliminate waste

To obtain this consistent motivation, compelling goals are needed. These include long-term and ambitious goals such as being the chair of a department by a certain date and short-term goals such as blocking away enough time during the day to complete all clinic notes without having to do any at home. We all need that psychological push to maintain discipline regarding scheduling and planning. Therefore, we should strive to create goals that create excitement and energy [12]. If not, one must strongly think about why he or she is setting that goal. We must remember it is okay to say no, and eliminating "waste", or tasks that do not achieve particular goals, often creates greater satisfaction for people in the long run.

Adopted from the industry, lean management has jumped to the forefront over the last decade as a service improvement technique in healthcare circles [13]. The overall premise is to identify and eliminate wasted resources, especially wasted time, by splitting up daily activities into three primary categories: (1) value-adding activities or ones that transform the service you deliver to meet the needs of your patients; (2) non-value-adding activities or ones that take your time and resources but do not add any value to the services you provide in the eyes of the patient; (3) necessary non-value-adding or activities that have to be carried out because they enable a value-adding activity or are a statutory requirement. Waste is any non-value-adding activity and/or poor use of time [14]. One of the largest time sinks for providers is wasted time spent waiting for people, documents, responses, or unnecessary travel while at work. In contrast, when one is finally able to focus on compelling goals while not getting bogged down with what may feel like meaningless tasks, motivation improves, as does productivity. By eliminating waste to streamline the completion of tasks in an efficient and satisfying manner that is consistent with closely held values, one can ultimately create a personal culture of productivity.

Strategies for Creating a Personal Culture of Productivity:

- Create compelling goals by reviewing your personal motivators.
- Highlight **value-adding activities** and try to eliminate **non-value-adding activities** in your daily routine.
- Write goals and motivators down as a reminder or share with a mentor or direct report for accountability.
- Don't be afraid to say no to tasks that are misaligned with values or goals.
- **Daily**: Review essential tasks to be accomplished today and by the end of the workweek.
- **Weekly**: Preview the upcoming week and prioritize key tasks.
- **Weekly**: Build in reminders to your calendar to complete tasks on time.
- **Monthly**: Evaluate recent points of failure or challenges in accomplishing goals.
- **Monthly**: Review all the things that have been accomplished and reflect on all the hard work you have done!
- **Quarterly**: Consider blocking out at least one day of protected time (nothing scheduled) for personal wellness or catching up on high-value tasks.
- **Annually**: Review 1, 5, and 10-year career goals and analyze areas where values and goals may need realignment.

Using Organization to Maintain Priorities

Much of the need to improve quality and deliver more efficient care in health systems stems from an organizational level. However, personal approaches to time management are essential, and creating well-constructed to-do lists can have a tremendous impact on minimizing a person's wasted time throughout the day to maintain priorities and complete value-added goals. These time management techniques can only develop in conjunction with other management skills such as priority setting, assertiveness, and delegation.

While to-do lists are all but essential in today's world, they are not effective on their own as a mere collection of random thoughts. These lists need to be prioritized, and as such, each item needs to be reviewed and ranked with regard to its priority. Furthermore, can the task be done by only you and does it have that sense of "must be done now" attached to it? President Dwight Eisenhower was one of the first to develop a personal time management system that divided tasks into four categories [2, 7]. This was later modified by Stephen Covey, most known for his book "The 7 Habits of Highly Effective People". In this book, he considers theoretically placing each task into one of four quadrants, prioritizing every aspect of work. Having sequenced these tasks into an order of priority, each person must then commit to action them [2, 7]. These categories can be modified to apply to urology.

- **Quadrant 1 tasks**—high urgency, high importance tasks including urologic emergencies, urgent clinic needs/patients, necessary and important meetings, deadline-driven projects, and last-minute preparations for scheduled activities.
- **Quadrant 2 tasks**—low urgency, high importance tasks: preparation/planning, wellness activities (exercise and social), grant writing, personal/career development tasks, research responsibilities, and preparing chapters.
- **Quadrant 3 tasks**—high urgency, low importance tasks: interruptions (pager going off, covering tasks for colleagues, and being asked to cover something just because you were walking through clinic), some mail and reports, some meetings, and many "pressing matters".
- **Quadrant 4 tasks**—low urgency, low importance tasks: many emails and phone calls, time sinks (social media and mindless television/Internet), busy work, and escape activities.

Consultants and trainees who spend most of their time working in quadrant 1 face burnout as they jump from one emergency or crisis to the next. The most effective people stay out of quadrants 3 and 4 and minimize the amount of time they spend tackling projects in quadrant 1. Instead, they optimize the time they spend working on quadrant 2, which allows them to gain better control and balance in their lives.

Complete "Quadrant 1" Tasks First: High Urgency, High Importance, Deadline-Driven

Urologists and medical professionals need to avoid spending every day reacting to unexpected events and dealing with one crisis after another. Though unavoidable at times, this style often compromises a healthy work-life balance. Therefore, once all quadrant 1 tasks have been identified, these should be dealt with first. One method of doing this is to set half an hour aside each week to schedule time to write out the tasks for the week, allowing one to effectively plan for the days ahead [2]. In the modern era, an electronic planner or calendar can also be synchronized with family members to provide a clear view of your commitments. This includes adding in all regular commitments such as surgeries, rounds, clinic schedules, meetings, and any appointments. Also, it is critical to schedule all quadrant 1 tasks as they must be finished in a timely fashion and should be focused on during the earlier part of the week, if possible.

When new to effective time management, it is also important to estimate how long one thinks a specific task will take and to schedule double that time. Poor time managers are notoriously erroneous when estimating the length of a task, and therefore, added time must be included until a person has a better idea of the true length of tasks [15]. By creating this habit of scheduling adequate time in your calendar for tasks every week, these number 1 tasks will be more easily eliminated. It is also important to know what time of day and part of the week one is the most efficient and to always protect this time. Performing these tasks during so-called "energy peaks" will allow tasks to get done more quickly [7]. For quadrant 2 tasks, which are hopefully the largest number of tasks on one's list, these should be scheduled throughout the week (think of a talk to be made for next month). In the beginning, it is best to start small by scheduling only a few of these each week to not get overwhelmed.

Learn to Say "NO"

Many in academia have ascended to success and subsequently increased responsibility due to the personality trait of reflexively saying yes. However, saying yes to everything (or at least most things) can present significant challenges to both efficiency and the quality of work one produces. Overcommitment can quickly mire a physician down into low-value, low-priority tasks and may lead to burnout. However, saying no often feels wrong due to perceived external perceptions or intrinsic assumptions of worthiness related to completing tasks when asked. Saying no effectively is one of the most useful tools for the busy urologist to ensure time for deep work as well as the pursuit of high-value and high-passion goals. Bruce Tulgan, writing in the Harvard Business Review Magazine, recommends a three-step process for assessing whether to say no to the many asks that may come, both formal and informal, within or external to your organization [16]. First, Tulgan recommends systematically evaluating the ask with the following questions:

1. When is the ask being made?
2. Who is the asker?
3. What deliverable is being requested (with specifics)?
4. What is the timeline?
5. What resources are needed?
6. Who is the source of authority, and is further permission needed to proceed?
7. What are possible benefits?
8. What are the obvious and hidden costs?

By considering these questions as soon as an ask for your time and efforts is made, you can develop a system for assessing the value of a proposition. Tulgan then recommends deciding and responding with either a "well-reasoned no" or an "effective yes". A well-reasoned no should be applied when something is not allowed, should not be pursued (either personally or corporately), or cannot be effectively completed. Timing is also important and a no should be delivered tactfully and respectfully to the asker, after careful consideration, and neither reflexively at the time of the ask, or in such a delayed fashion that one seems negligent. In contrast, according to Tulgan, an effective yes is,

> ...aligned with the mission, values, priorities, ground rules, and marching orders from above. It's for something that you can do, ideally well, fast, and with confidence. In other words, it involves one of your specialties—or an opportunity to build a new one.

Nevertheless, even with a systematic way to evaluate opportunities, saying no is still often exceedingly difficult. Here are some considerations for how to say no differently, summarized from an excellent article from *INC. Magazine* on "7 Tips for Saying No Effectively" [17]. The author, Jonathan Alpert, recommends the following actions when saying no:

1. **Say it**. Anything short of verbalizing or writing NO is potentially considered a yes.
2. **Be courteous and assertive**.
3. **Understand peoples' tactics**. Recognize when manipulation techniques or social pressures may be utilized to try to get you to say yes when you really mean no.
4. **Set Boundaries**.
5. **Put the question back on the person asking**. If a timeline or a request conflicts with a known obligation, ask how the conflicting tasks should be prioritized which may lead to a nullification of the unrealistic request.
6. **Stand Firm**. If someone will not accept a well-reasoned no, they are signaling their priorities in the work relationship.
7. **Be Selfish**. Sometimes you must put your own needs first to protect your most important priorities.

Granted, saying no is not easy, but utilizing techniques for saying no when appropriate will preserve personal time and capital to make important contributions that align with your values. Saying no may become one of your most effective tools for time management within the domain of setting priorities.

Section 2: Minimizing Distractions

Distractions abound in a busy academic center. Whether the everpresent unexpected patient urgency or emergency or the well-meaning colleague who finds a way to derail your plans for focused work, minimizing the impact of distractions is paramount to succeeding in a bustling workplace. The second section of this chapter focuses on techniques for minimizing distractions.

What Do I Do All Day?

Understanding how your time is being spent is the first step to minimizing distractions. Each person should spend some time in introspection to determine the best part of the day or night that allows focused completion of tasks. These tasks may be an upcoming book chapter, grant proposals, the annual Holiday letter, recommendation letters for colleagues, or medical charts. Scheduling in advance during that time to complete tasks for upcoming deadlines aids in completing tasks without the last-minute scramble that many have endured. Conversely, identifying times when focused work is very difficult (such as on-call or immediately after a physically or emotionally taxing clinic) is also important to design periods of productivity into the surgeon's routine.

Taking time to speak and relax with friends and family every single day for at least a short period is also essential to recharge and improve focus on responsibilities for the remainder of the day. The same goes for allowing periods of contemplation/reflection, engagement in social media, and completion of "9 to 5" business such as scheduling personal appointments external to work. As part of this budgeted time, one should also strive to exercise frequently as physical health also serves to improve mental stamina and acumen and prolong a busy surgeon's career by avoiding chronic injury. Determining what you do during a regular day, week, month, or as part of the larger seasons of life will then allow you to schedule focused work effectively.

Schedule Gaps in Your day

For better or worse, unforeseen events or emergencies will always interrupt the normal workflow of a day. Although unexpected, these can also be planned for by not scheduling every day with back-to-back meetings or appointments. Leaving gaps in every working day not only provides for breathing space but allows for the time to deal with something potentially unexpected [18]. Most importantly, this can alleviate stress by still allowing for unexpected quadrant 1 tasks to be completed. Using your understanding of when you work best and then scheduling gaps during that time is a powerful combination to ensure productivity.

When multi-tasking cannot be avoided, it is key to perform each task effectively while avoiding doing a poor job at any of them. The importance of the tasks and what they require followed by balancing the attention and effort that the simultaneous tasks require is essential. For example, while on hold and waiting to speak to a patient's family after surgery, a surgeon can have the patient's electronic chart open to complete the operative note and complete various electronic signatures that are required during this forced downtime. Learning what tasks can and cannot successfully be performed in combination will allow you to leverage greater productivity in the long run.

   In addition to scheduling gaps in their daily schedule, some physicians find it useful to schedule a weekday of time-off each quarter or at least twice a year. This ensures some built-in protected time that can then be used as a day to catch up since nothing will be scheduled to conflict. This can allow an unexpected, but useful break to deal with pressing issues that have accumulated. If there are no tasks to be completed when this protected day arrives, then a true day off can be enjoyed! More will be discussed about protected time in the next section.

Protected Time and Importance of "Protecting Protected Time"

Though difficult for many to acknowledge, it is okay to be assertive and say no, and it is also ok to use physical distance or other barriers to protect focused work. While planning for an organization is part of the equation, one must also prioritize protecting their own time. After one identifies when he or she is most productive, this person must also find ways to minimize interruptions that occur during this block. For example, during this protected time, one can ignore the telephone and/or set their email inbox to "offline". Most cellular phones now have a customizable "do not disturb" function that allows you to set a privileged list of designated callers whose calls or texts will connect if in "do not disturb mode" (i.e., chief resident, boss, or spouse). Consider leveraging such technology to allow minimal interruptions during specific times. If this protected time is during the day, consider shutting the door and placing a note that says to only knock if it is an emergency. Furthermore, always have projects available that one can do in small parcels of time. If one prefers to procrastinate or if a task feels so overwhelming he or she does not know where to begin, try breaking the task into smaller pieces that can be scheduled over a period. This "salami principle", or cutting big projects into slices, allows for consistent progress to be made each week to hit a deadline. By eating the slices one at a time, one will eventually consume the entire salami (i.e., project) [19].

Finding Time for Yourself Will Improve Your Work Focus

A guide to Self-help on the National Health Service (NHS) website states the aim of good time management is to achieve the lifestyle balance you want. This work-life balance is "achieved when an individual's right to a fulfilled life inside and outside paid work is accepted and respected as the norm, to the mutual benefit of the individual, business, and society" [20]. These benefits transcend all levels of the individual's life, given positive mental health is associated with decreased absences from work, a more positive work culture, and improved recruitment and retention.

Fig. 15.1 The wheel of life

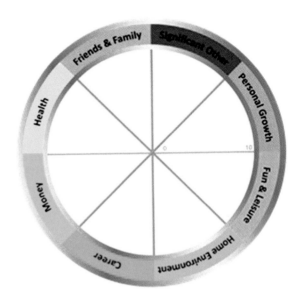

Altogether, benefits include improved job satisfaction and better satisfaction with family life, both of which can yield more energy and enthusiasm within the workforce. Perceived competence is improved as well. Therefore, it is essential to find time to do those things you love outside of work.

One exercise that can help balance the multiple needs we all have is called the "wheel of life" [7, 21]. This personal development tool allows for a visual representation of one's life balance and is made up of eight sections (Fig. 15.1).

Instructions:

- Imagine a scale from 0–10, with a 0 at the center of the circle and a 10 at the periphery of each segment.
- Grade your current level of satisfaction with each segment by drawing a dot to create a new outer edge, then join each dot up to create a new perimeter. If you are very satisfied with a particular area of your life, it would be rated 9 or 10 out of 10; if there are areas of your life where you have not accomplished what you want or it is not bringing the satisfaction you hoped for, give it a lower rating.
- The new perimeter of the circle represents your current balance wheel.

Reflective questions

- What did you score and why? Would this score have been consistent a year ago? Three years ago? And are we happy with these changes?
- Which segment do you feel needs to be improved the most? Is there one segment that if improved, would result in others being improved?
- Ask yourself, what area/s do I want to improve the most on? Am I focusing too much time on one area?

Limiting Social Media and Unnecessary Internet Usage

The Internet undoubtedly speeds up staying in communication with employees, patients, and colleagues and facilitates research, but unnecessary use can present distractions to the workflow of an office [22]. To maximize efficiency, one must try to limit their use of social media and other websites of minimal value. One easy method to accomplish this is to monitor your online patterns to determine whether you are focusing on the tasks that matter most to the practice. Web-based time tracking and time monitoring tools can help track the amount of time spent emailing and the frequency with which certain websites are visited. There are also ways to block visiting certain websites at work (Gmail, Facebook, Twitter, etc.) to further minimize unnecessary distractions [23]. A study by Michael Porter that tracked 27 CEOs over 3 months found these CEOs spent 24% of their time simply replying to emails, many of which were unnecessary. Resultantly, these CEOs were often pulled into the operational weeds when they did not need to be. As Porter stated, "E-mail interrupts works, extends the workday, intrudes on family and thinking, and is not conducive to thoughtful discussions. CEOs have to stay human and authentic, and you can't do that via email" [23].

Key Takeaways:

- Audit utilization of non-work websites and applications by setting your phone or computer to track usage.
- Review usage patterns:

    - time spent on distractions,
    - most-visited or used applications/sites, and
    - the number of times checking email.

- If you find yourself lacking the self-discipline to limit social media or Internet usage, utilize technology to impose limits.
- Budget time for social media or Internet browsing during specified times.
- Develop a system for when to check and respond to emails to maintain boundaries.

Additional pearls for minimizing distractions and improving performance

A frequent complaint from managers and employees is that workers often spend their days in a state of constant distraction and task switching. This results in people being busy but not necessarily productive. More than a quarter of the time when someone switches tasks, it is two hours or more before they may resume what they were previously doing. Altogether, these distractions take a toll. Employees who manage attention poorly are often in reactive mode, preventing them from being able to reflect and thoughtfully apply their knowledge or experience in a maximally efficient manner—the main reason they were hired in the first place [2]. Although everyone has a distinct set of ideas on how to maximize productivity, the following is a list of pearls we strongly abide by to maximize one's time.

Pareto principle (the 80:20 rule)

80% of one's time-consuming activities are generated by 20% of the causes, which usually stem from people or unresolved situations [24]. Here, it can be highly rewarding to invest the time to address a situation such as having that difficult conversation with an employee who is always interrupting your protected time to talk during the day. This principle also pertains to many other aspects of work including delegation, where it may prove beneficial to invest time in the training or development of someone to do some of your tasks. The same can be said of 20% of workers contributing approximately 80% of the results. By focusing on rewarding those high-performers and improving their retention rate, one can make drastic improvements.

Limit transition time

This pertains to the time spent commuting or waiting, as some people will spend substantial periods of their day walking from rounds to surgery to the clinic and to meetings. Without realizing it, this can greatly affect one's productivity. Therefore, finding ways to consolidate movement and the locations of meetings can help tremendously. The utilization of virtual meetings has helped improve transition times significantly in the modern workplace.

Keep the workspace clean and organized

Though it sounds simple, enjoying the aesthetics of your workplace can increase productivity by making one more inclined to work at a particular location. Make it a routine to tidy up at least weekly to keep your workspace organized.

Exercise and practice physical wellness

Performing surgery is a physical task and surgeons are at risk for career-threatening occupational injuries [25–28]. Among even minimally invasive surgeons and endoscopists, 60–86% reported physical pain related to the performance of their work. However, exercise, surgical microbreaks, and good sleep all seem to be protective factors [25–28]. Interestingly, taking short breaks during a long procedure (>2 h) does not seem to prolong overall surgical time [28]. Audit your weekly routine and make time for exercise and adequate rest to ensure vitality on the back half of your career. Your career depends upon it.

Abide by the 4 "D's" of decision-making.

- Does this task need to be done? If not, delete it.
- Do I need to do it? If not, delegate it.
- Do I need to do it now? If not, put it in your calendar for a future time/date.
- Do it now. If the task has arrived and needs to be done now, do it as such.

Batching

Dedicate blocks of time to similar tasks, i.e., emails and phone calls, reviewing electronic medical record to-dos, and notifying patients of test results.

Conclusion

As urologists and most medical providers can attest, the number of competing demands for our time is increasing more than ever, bringing good time management skills to the center of numerous training and coaching seminars. While there is not one general recipe that applies to everyone, the purpose of this review is to provide salient strategies that the reader may find applicable to adopt into their everyday life. As Stephen Covey eloquently stated, "By centering our lives on correct principles and creating a balanced focus between doing and increasing our ability to do, we become empowered in the task of creating effective, useful, and peaceful lives…for ourselves, and for our posterity".[2] Few of us need to radically overthrow our organizational culture overnight, but instead should consider incremental changes. Interestingly, the missing piece is often to say no instead of yes to protect that which is most important in our day-to-day pursuits. By adopting small and impactful changes over time, one can slowly and deliberately improve organizational effectiveness, and in turn, enjoy a profoundly positive impact on quality of life.

Financial support and sponsorship: Woodson W. Smelser, MD was supported by the Ruth L. Kirchenstein Institutional National Research Service Award (T32) Grant.

References

1. Alighieri D. The divine comedy.
2. Covey SR. The 7 habits of highly effective people: powerful lessons in personal change. New York: Simon and Schuster; 2004.
3. Twenge JM. Time period and birth cohort differences in depressive symptoms in the U.S., 1982–2013. Soc Indic Res. 2015;121(2):437–54.
4. Norful A, Rosenfeld A, Schroeder K. Travers J. Aliyu S. Primary drivers and psychological manifestations of stress in frontline healthcare workforce during the initial COVID-19 outbreak in the United States. Gen Hosp Psychiatry. 2021;69:20–26.
5. The mental health of health care workers in COVID-19: Results of The Healthcare Worker Sruvey. Mental Health America. 2021 Online. https://mhanational.org/mental-health-healthcare-workers-covid-19
6. Franklin B, Conrad C. The Way to Wealth: Ben Franklin on money and success. 2011. Createspace Independent Publishing Platform.
7. Birnie A, Caygill P, Hobkirk M. A time management guide for urologists. Urology News. 2016;20(5):1–4.

8. Thirteen important moments in the history of management. Business Insider. https://www.businessinsider.com/13-important-moments-in-the-history-of-time-management-2011-6

9. Snow R. I invented the modern age: the rise of Henry Ford. 2014. Simon and Schuster.

10. McCay JT, Ward R, and Ward LB. The management of time. Prentice Hall; 1958.

11. Zeratsky J. To get more done, focus on environment, expectations, and examples. 2018. https://hbr.org/2018/11/to-get-more-done-focus-on-environment-expectations-and-examples

12. Allen D. Getting things done: the art of stress-free productivity. A Penguin Book; 2015.

13. Campbell RJ. Thinking lean in healthcare. J AHIMA. 2009;80(6):40–3.

14. Tsasis P, Bruce-Barrett C. Organizational change through lean thinking. Health Serv Manage Res. 2008;21(2):192.

15. Robbins T. The ultimate guide to time management. https://www.tonyrobbins.com/importance-time-management/.

16. Learn when to say no. Harvard Business Review. https://hbr.org/2020/09/learn-when-to-say-no.

17. Alpert J. 7 Tips for Saying No Effectively. Inc. Magazine. https://www.inc.com/jonathan-alpert/7-ways-to-say-no-to-someone-and-not-feel-bad-about-it.html.

18. Ferriss T. The 4-hour workweek. 2007. Crown Publishing Group.

19. Bliss EC, Howey C. Getting Things Done: The ABCs of Time Management. The CEO Refresher. http://www.refresher.com/!chhtime.html.

20. NHS time management tips. http://www.nhs.uk/conditions/stress-anxiety-depression/pages/time-management-tips.aspx.

21. Williams JA (2014) Super training guide: academic life coaching's training program. Academic Life Coaching: Portland, OR.

22. Belsky S. 5 ways to reduce social media distractions and be more productive. https://mashable.com/2010/04/15/reduce-social-media-distractions/#WFvZ9jJ.hkqA.

23. Porter ME, Nohria N. How CEOs manage time. https://hbr.org/2018/07/the-leaders-calendar.

24. Kock R. The 80/20 principle: the secret to achieving more with less. Currency; 1999.

25. Harvin G. Review of musculoskeletal injuries and prevention in the endoscopy practitioner. J Clin Gastroenterol. 2014;48(7):590–4.

26. Sari V, Nieboer T, Vierhout M, et al. The operation room as a hostile environment for surgeons: physical complaints during and after laparoscopy. Minim Invasive Ther Allied Technol. 2010;19(2):105–9.

27. Park A, Lee G, Seagull F, et al. Patients benefit while surgeons suffer: an impending epidemic. J Am Coll Surg. 2010;210(3):306–13.

28. Hallbeck M, Lowndes B, Bingener J, et al. The impact of intraoperative microbreaks with exercises on surgeons: a multi-center cohort study. Appl Ergon. 2017;60:334–41.

Chapter 16
Media and Social Media

Stacy Loeb

Types of Social Media Platforms

Public Platforms

Numerous public-facing social media platforms are currently available. Some of the most popular platforms include Facebook, Instagram, Twitter, YouTube, and LinkedIn. Facebook is a social networking platform started in 2004, which allows users to post comments, share photos or videos, and send messages with other users. Instagram is a photo and video-sharing social network that was launched in 2010. Twitter is a microblogging platform which was launched in 2006, and allows users to communicate through short messages called tweets (originally limited to 140 characters, but subsequently increased to 280 characters). YouTube is a widely used video-sharing platform launched in 2005, and LinkedIn is a professional, business-oriented social network that was founded in 2002. Other public-facing social media platforms include TikTok (short-form videos) and Pinterest (sharing of images and other information).

The major professional societies in urology, such as the American Urological Association and the European Association of Urology, have a presence on multiple social media platforms (e.g., Facebook, Twitter, YouTube, etc.). Social media are also widely used by urological patients for a variety of reasons. For example, there are many communities on Facebook and other online discussion forums for patients and their families with a variety of urologic conditions (e.g. exstrophy, sexual dysfunction, genitourinary cancer). Many advocacy groups and foundations also have social media pages with patient education materials (e.g. Urology Care Foundation). The majority of urologists also actively participate in social media.

S. Loeb (✉)
Department of Urology and Population Health, New York University and Manhattan Veterans Affairs, 227 E 30th Street #612, New York, NY 10016, USA
e-mail: stacyloeb@gmail.com

A survey of American Urological Association members in 2017 reported that 74% had a social media account [1]. Facebook was the most commonly used social media platform by urologists, although there were significant increases in the use of LinkedIn, Twitter, Instagram, and Pinterest over time.

Platforms for Healthcare Professionals

In addition to the public-facing platforms described above, there are several social media platforms specifically for healthcare professionals. One of these is Doximity, which allows physicians and other healthcare professionals (e.g., nurse practitioners and physician assistants) to create their own profile and to network with each other. The Doximity app also offers other services for healthcare providers, such as a news feed with relevant articles, tracking of continuing medical education activity, a secure fax, and the "Doximity Dialer" to facilitate phone or video calls to patients. In addition, Doximity currently serves as the exclusive provider for online physician surveys used in U.S. News and World Report. Sermo is another social media platform directed at physicians. The goal of Sermo is to connect physicians with the support and wisdom of their peers. It has several different features including medical news, case-based discussions, polls, and drug ratings. Sermo also offers paid surveys for physicians for medical market research.

Urology-Specific Social Media Guidelines

There are multiple social media guidelines and best practice statements specific for urologists, which were recently reviewed [2]. Before engaging with social media, it is recommended that all urologists and trainees familiarize themselves with these recommendations to ensure appropriate use according to professional standards.

One of these is the Social Media Best Practices by the American Urological Association [3]. The key points are to be professional, courteous, and thoughtful; to protect confidentiality and exercise discretion; to allow for interaction; and to support the identity of the AUA.

The British Journal of Urology International (BJUI) also has guidelines on Engaging Responsibly with Social Media [4]. They recommend always considering that your content will exist forever and be available to everyone. If you are a doctor, you should identify yourself; however, you should state that your views are your own if your institutions are identifiable. You should also maintain a professional boundary between you and your patients, and protect patient's privacy and confidentiality at all times. Your digital profile and behavior online must align with the standards of your profession, you should avoid impropriety, disclose potential conflicts of interest, always be truthful, and strive for accuracy. They also recommend not to post content in anger and to alert colleagues if you feel they have posted the content which may be deemed inappropriate for a doctor.

The European Association of Urology recently issued updated Recommendations on the Appropriate Use of Social Media, including 10 key points: (1) Understand how other users behave online before interacting on social networks; (2) Establish and maintain a professional digital identity that is in line with your professional practice and goals; (3) Never undermine your patients' privacy or confidentiality; (4) Avoid providing medical advice and maintain limits between yourself and patients; (5) Assume that anything and everything you post is permanent; (6) Use instant messaging services with care; (7) Exercise professionalism; (8) Beware of social media policies set by employers; (9) Beware of how advertisement and self-promotion will be perceived by others; and (10) Use disease-specific hashtags for structured online communication [5]. Many other medical societies have guidance regarding online behavior, and it is also important to familiarize yourself with the policy at your own institution prior to active use.

Benefits of Social Media

There are many ways in which social media can benefit the practicing urologist. In a 2014 survey of users participating in Twitter during the AUA and EAU meetings, 97% of respondents agreed that Twitter is useful for networking [6]. In addition, 96%, 75%, 74%, and 62% of respondents agreed that it is useful for disseminating information, research, advocacy, and career development.

Clinical Practice

Social media are a useful way to advertise your clinical practice. Many individual urologists, urology practices, academic departments, and hospitals have a presence on social media (e.g., Facebook pages, YouTube videos, etc.). Particularly in light of the large number of third-party websites with ratings of physicians, it is important to monitor your online presence on an ongoing basis. Individual pages on Facebook, Twitter, and other public-facing social media platforms typically rank highly in online searches, and therefore maintaining an active presence can increase the probability that your own content appears at the top of a search.

For urology departments, greater Twitter activity (e.g., more followers and higher Klout scores) has a significant correlation with U.S. News and World Report reputation scores [7]. Although it is not possible to establish a causal relationship, it seems likely that social media promotions can enhance the reputation of urology departments and individual urologists.

In addition, social media are also being used by individual urologists for crowdsourcing of cases. Recent publications have demonstrated the use of social media platforms to discuss specific cases, leading to actual changes in patient management [8]. A 2014 survey of active urological Twitter users reported that 44% of physicians agreed it was useful for clinical decision-making and 33% had made a clinical decision after a Twitter discussion [6].

Research

Social media can be used at multiple stages of research in urology. First, it may be used for research recruitment. Numerous studies have used social media platforms such as Facebook and Twitter for recruitment of urological patients and/or healthcare providers for research studies [6, 9]. Social media can also be used for as a source of data for research. For example, previous studies have used Twitter data as a barometer for public interest and sentiment about particular topics, such as major changes in clinical guidelines [10]. Other studies have examined the quality of information about urological conditions being shared on social platforms (e.g. YouTube, TikTok) [11–13].

Finally, social media is a useful tool for research dissemination. All of the major journals maintain an active presence on social media. Some urology journals request authors to write a tweet about their paper as part of the submission process. This can later be used to promote the dissemination of papers once published, which is beneficial for both the researchers and the journal.

Due to the importance of online research dissemination, many journals have recently begun converting the key points of new publications into ˜visual abstracts' that can be readily shared on social media. Studies in the surgical literature have demonstrated that tweeting a visual abstract significantly increases the reach of tweets and the number of article visits, compared to only tweeting the title of new papers [14].

Studies have shown that having a Twitter presence is associated with impact factor for urological journals [15], and is associated with citations for individual urology papers [16]. It seems logical that greater social media activity surrounding a publication helps to spread the research among a broader audience, thereby increasing the potential for citations and hopefully also increasing the probability that the evidence therein will positively impact patient care.

Education

Social media can also be a useful source for education. A survey of urology trainees in Europe revealed that YouTube was the preferred platform for learning about surgical technique, more so than textbooks or journal articles [17]. Although these platforms can be extremely useful to share educational content with a wide audience, quality control is extremely important. For example, a previous study of YouTube videos about mid-urethral slings found that many were missing key steps of the operation [12].

Social media are also widely used at urological conferences. It is possible to follow along with conference proceedings through the dedicated social media feed.

Although some content about urological conferences is frequently posted on multiple different social platforms (e.g., Facebook, LinkedIn), Twitter provides the most expedient platform to follow the proceedings in real-time. Each of the major urological meetings has its own hashtag (or metadata tag), which is typically an abbreviation combining the name of the meeting and the year (e.g., #AUA22, #EAU22). Some conferences also have physical Twitter boards in public areas, or screens on the podium showing the Twitter feed so that moderators can incorporate questions from viewers into the discussion. Since many conferences have multiple sessions occurring simultaneously, following the conference hashtag on Twitter can provide a useful supplement to the experience. Social media also enables remote participation in conferences for those who cannot attend in person. In a 2014 survey of urological Twitter users, 76% indicated that they had followed a congress remotely [6]. In this way, social networks can enhance the conference experience and facilitate global sharing of knowledge.

Social media are also a useful way to stay up-to-date with clinical practice guidelines. Beginning in 2014, the European Association of Urology Guidelines Office initiated a project to convert the key points from all of its urology guidelines into tweets for public dissemination [18]. During the first 18 months of this experience, tweets about the EAU guidelines reached an audience of >9 million. This demonstrates the potential for social media to promote evidence-based practice in urology.

There are also multiple Twitter-based journal clubs which allow global discussions of important new research [19]. The first of these efforts in urology was the International Urology Journal Club (#urojc). Since that time, other Twitter-based journal clubs have been initiated such as the Pediatric Urology Journal Club (#pedurojc) and Prostate Cancer Journal Club (#prostatejc) [20, 21].

Finally, social media can be used for patient education and outreach. As described above, many urological patients are using social media platforms to network with each other and discuss healthcare. Involvement in social media provides a vast audience for urologists to contribute to public education and engage with patients. For example, some urologists maintain YouTube channels or blogs with educational information for patients, which can also increase visibility and help to recruit new patients to your practice.

Drawbacks to Social Media

One of the pitfalls of social media as a source of information is that there is a large quantity of user-generated content that has not been vetted. Previous studies have evaluated the quality of online information about various urological conditions on social media, with sobering results. Important considerations include readability, understandability, actionability, and representation of racial and ethnic diversity [22]. Studies of content about urological issues on multiple social networks have identified information that is written above the recommended reading level for consumer health information, uses jargon, or does not otherwise provide information that is easily actionable for lay audiences.

Another major issue is spread of misinformation. A recent study examined the top 150 YouTube videos about prostate cancer and found that 77% contained potentially misinformative or biased content in the video itself or the comments section underneath it [11]. Concerningly, there was a significant inverse relationship between the expert-rated scientific quality of the videos and the amount of user engagement (i.e., lower quality videos had a greater number of views and thumbs up from viewers). Studies of online content about other urological conditions have similarly reported the presence of misinformative content [12]. Several other studies have similarly demonstrated the spread of misinformation about a variety of urological conditions on different social networks, which were recently reviewed [23]. To help mitigate this, urologists should recommend trusted resources for patients and their families to obtain additional information outside the medical encounter. In addition, urologists should actively participate in social media and post high-quality content to help raise the signal above the noise.

Another potential risk of social media for urologists and other healthcare providers is professional misconduct. Studies of urology trainees and junior faculty have suggested the presence of potentially unprofessional content on publicly visible Facebook pages [24]. Although there are several urology-specific guidelines on professional social media use, recent global surveys of urologists and trainees indicated that approximately 2/3 were not familiar with them, despite that the majority participate in these networks [25, 26]. The importance of following these recommendations cannot be understated and all urologists planning to use social media should review them.

Finally, excessive social media participation can have other psychological and physical consequences. In fact, social media disorder is now recognized as an emerging mental health problem, leading to the development of multiple scales to measure addiction to social media [27]. Recent surveys have reported that a small proportion of urologists and trainees meet the criteria for social media disorder [25, 26].

In terms of physical impact, most urologists view social media using smartphones. Excessive time bending over a smartphone in a forward flexed neck position may lead to musculoskeletal problems including increased neck pain ("text neck") and possibly a greater risk of disk degeneration [28]. Overall, moderate use in accordance with professional guidelines is the best approach to maximize the benefits and reduce risks.

Conventional Media

Practicing urologists may also be interested in becoming involved with conventional media, such as TV, radio, or print media. To get started, consider your goals and what you hope to accomplish through media involvement (e.g., public education, advertising for your practice, etc.) and the type of media that you would like to participate in. If you work for a hospital or university, contact the media department at your institution to express an interest in getting involved. Some physicians also work with a publicist to help increase their exposure and book relevant media opportunities.

If you have important information to share, you (or your publicist) can make a pitch to producers/editors at the desired media outlets. A pitch can be done through email, briefly summarizing your relevant expertise and what you can uniquely share with the audience. Participating actively in social media is also a great way to connect with the media organically.

For urologists involved in scientific publications, it is important to maintain an ongoing relationship with the media department at your institution about works in progress and keep them notified well in advance if an important research paper will be published. If the findings hold great public interest, the media department can issue a press release, which will greatly increase the visibility of your research. It is important to carefully review the content of the press release, since excerpts from this are often shared by multiple media outlets.

When contacted by the media to participate in an interview, it is important to respond promptly to these inquiries. For live or taped interviews with public-facing media outlets, remember to use lay language and avoid medical jargon. For print media, there are often strict deadlines so it is important to provide the desired content in a timely fashion. Producers, editors, writers, and hosts will remember experts who do a great job and respond promptly. These relationships are essential for urologists seeking repeated, ongoing media opportunities.

Key Points

- Social media are widely used by medical societies, healthcare providers, patients, and other stakeholders.
- There are multiple public-facing social networks as well as platforms specific to healthcare professionals.
- The majority of urologists have a social media account.
- Social media has many potential benefits for clinical care, research, and education.
- Social media has potential risks including the spread of misinformation and professional misconduct.
- Urologists should review the professional guidelines on social media prior to use.
- Maintain an ongoing relationship with your institution's media department to identify potential opportunities.
- Respond to media inquiries promptly and avoid using medical jargon during interviews.

References

1. Loeb S, Carrick T, Frey C, Titus T. Increasing social media use in urology: 2017 American urological association survey. Eur Urol Focus. 2020;6:605–8.
2. Taylor J, Loeb S. Guideline of guidelines: social media in urology. BJU Int. 2020;125:379–82.
3. American Urological Association Social Media Best Practices. http://auanet.mediaroom.com/index.php?s=20294. Accessed 30 Sept 2018.
4. Murphy DG, Loeb S, Basto MY, Challacombe B, Trinh QD, Leveridge M, et al. Engaging responsibly with social media: the BJUI guidelines. BJU Int. 2014;114:9–11.
5. Borgmann H, Cooperberg M, Murphy D, Loeb S, N'Dow J, Ribal MJ, et al. Online professionalism-2018 update of European Association of Urology (@Uroweb) recommendations on the appropriate use of social media. Eur Urol. 2018. S0302-2838(18)30614-6. https://doi.org/10.1016/j.eururo.2018.08.022.
6. Borgmann H, DeWitt S, Tsaur I, Haferkamp A, Loeb S. Novel survey disseminated through Twitter supports its utility for networking, disseminating research, advocacy, clinical practice and other professional goals. Can Urol Assoc J. 2015;9:E713–7.
7. Ciprut S, Curnyn C, Davuluri M, Sternberg K, Loeb S. Twitter activity associated With US news and world report reputation scores for urology departments. Urology. 2017;108:11–6.
8. Sternberg KM, Loeb SL, Canes D, Donnelly L, Tsai MH. The use of Twitter to facilitate sharing of clinical expertise in urology. J Am Med Inform Assoc. 2018;25:183–6.
9. Rowe CK, Shnorhavorian M, Block P, Ahn J, Merguerian PA. Using social media for patient-reported outcomes: A study of genital appearance and sexual function in adult bladder exstrophy patients. J Pediatr Urol. 2018;14(322):e1–6.
10. Prabhu V, Lee T, Loeb S, Holmes JH, Gold HT, Lepor H, et al. Twitter response to the United States preventive services task force recommendations against screening with prostate-specific antigen. BJU Int. 2015;116:65–71.
11. Loeb S, Sengupta S, Butaney M, Macaluso JN, Jr., Czarniecki SW, Robbins R, et al. Dissemination of misinformative and biased information about prostate Cancer on YouTube. Eur Urol. 2018.
12. Larouche M, Geoffrion R, Lazare D, Clancy A, Lee T, Koenig NA, et al. Mid-urethral slings on YouTube: quality information on the internet? Int Urogynecol J. 2016;27:903–8.
13. Xu AJ, Taylor J, Gao T, Mihalcea R, Perez-Rosas V, Loeb S. TikTok and prostate cancer: misinformation and quality of information using validated questionnaires. BJU Int. 2021. https://doi.org/10.1111/bju.15403.
14. Ibrahim AM, Lillemoe KD, Klingensmith ME, Dimick JB. Visual abstracts to disseminate research on social media: a prospective, case-control crossover study. Annals Surg. 2017;266: e46–8.
15. Nason GJ, O'Kelly F, Kelly ME, Phelan N, Manecksha RP, Lawrentschuk N, et al. The emerging use of Twitter by urological journals. BJU Int. 2015;115:486–90.
16. Hayon S, Tripathi H, Stormont IM, Dunne MM, Naslund MJ, Siddiqui MM. Twitter mentions and academic citations in the urologic literature. Urology. 2018.
17. Rivas JG, Socarras MR, Patruno G, Uvin P, Esperto F, Dinis PJ, et al. Perceived role of social media in urologic knowledge acquisition among young urologists: A European survey. Eur Urol Focus. 2018;4:768–73.
18. Loeb S, Roupret M, Van Oort I, N'Dow J, van Gurp M, Bloemberg J, et al. Novel use of Twitter to disseminate and evaluate adherence to clinical guidelines by the European Association of Urology. BJU Int. 2017;119:820–2.
19. Topf JM, Sparks MA, Phelan PJ, Shah N, Lerma EV, Graham-Brown MPM, et al. The evolution of the journal club: from Osler to Twitter. Am J Kidney Dis. 2017;69:827–36.
20. Truong H, Salib A, Rowe CK. The use of social media in pediatric urology-forging new paths or crossing boundaries? Curr Urol Rep. 2019;20:72.

21. Loeb S, Taylor J, Butaney M, Byrne NK, Gao L, Soule HR, et al. Twitter-based Prostate Cancer Journal Club (#ProstateJC) Promotes multidisciplinary global scientific discussion and research dissemination. Eur Urol. 2019;75:881–2.
22. Borno HT, Zhang S, Bakke B, Bell A, Zuniga KB, Li P, et al. Racial disparities and online health information: YouTube and prostate cancer clinical trials. BJU Int. 2020;126:11–3.
23. Loeb S, Taylor J, Borin JF, Mihalcea R, Perez-Rosas V, Byrne N, et al. Fake news: spread of misinformation about urological conditions on social media. Eur Urol Focus. 2019;6:437–9.
24. Koo K, Bowman MS, Ficko Z, Gormley EA. Older and wiser? Changes in unprofessional content on urologists' social media after transition from residency to practice. BJU Int. 2018;122:337–43.
25. Dubin JM, Greer AB, Patel P, Carrion DM, Paesano N, Kettache RH, et al. Global survey of the roles and attitudes toward social media platforms amongst urology trainees. Urology. 2021;147:64–7.
26. Dubin JM, Greer AB, Patel P, Carrion DM, Paesano N, Kettache RH, et al. Global survey evaluating drawbacks of social media usage for practising urologists. BJU Int. 2020;126:7–8.
27. van den Eijnden RJJM, Lemmens JS, Valkenburg PM. The Social Media Disorder Scale. Comput Hum Behav. 2016;61:478–87.
28. Cuellar JM, Lanman TH. "Text neck": an epidemic of the modern era of cell phones? Spine J Off J North Am Spine Soc. 2017;17:901–2.

Chapter 17
Burnout, Happiness and Work-Life Harmony

Granville L. Lloyd and Sarah E. McAchran

Introduction

How can one achieve success, in urology or anything, and still preserve "balance" in life? Is balance a goal that is commensurate with success, or are the two inherently at odds with each other? Can one achieve success in urology without making sacrifices? How can my career best be used as a vehicle for happiness, fulfillment and self-expression?

For all of us that survived residency, it is clear that sacrifice and hard work are required to achieve basic competence, let alone success. Those that continue to pursue success after such an ordeal, whether via the endless work of academics or the high-volume grindstone of a busy private practice would never deny the hard work required. To quote Dean Simonton, a psychology professor who has studied success at length: "People who wish (success) must organize their whole lives around a single enterprise. They must be monomaniacs, even megalomaniacs, about their pursuits. They must start early, labor continuously, and never give up the cause" [1].

If that sounds awful… well, that's why you're here. Is the goal of life, start to finish, to merely survive? To claw one's way through Maslow's hierarchical needs? To make a lasting contribution and see your statue erected at your home institution? To laser a couple stones and make it to the club by 3? Those goals, such as they may be, need to be identified and pursued differently in each person, and yours probably vary more from the person in the next office than you suspect. But where

G. L. Lloyd (✉)
UC Health at University of Colorado Anschutz Medical Campus, Aurora, CO 80045, USA
e-mail: granville.lloyd@CUAnschutz.edu

Department of Surgery/ Urology, Rocky Mountain Regional VA, Aurora, USA

S. E. McAchran
Dyad Lead, UW Medical Foundation Centennial Building, 1685 Highland Avenue, Madison, WI 53705-2281, USA

© The Author(s), under exclusive license to Springer Nature Switzerland AG 2022   171
S. Y. Nakada and S. R. Patel (eds.), *Navigating Organized Urology*,
https://doi.org/10.1007/978-3-031-05540-9_17

does work fit in to that for you? Is "work" really something counter to "life" such that one needs less of one to achieve the other in order to achieve balance?

This chapter argues no. Work, if nothing more than a means of managing that pesky mortgage bill that arrives each month, sounds mundane at best and awful on average. You have chosen a profession, an art and science; a calling: fight to prevent it from deteriorating into less. Work devoid of meaning and purpose leads to burnout. The Maslach Burnout Index (MBI) assesses three distinct components of burnout: emotional exhaustion, depersonalization, and personal accomplishment/experience of ineffectiveness [2]. Aside from the personal, psychological toll burnout takes, burnt out physicians are associated with decreased quality of care, decreased patient satisfaction, increased medical errors, and increased staff turnover [3].

Along with teaching and law, medicine is one of the "noble professions," and as such has the chance to achieve that holy grail of work: personal meaning and fulfillment. When you are able to connect to work, or to craft work to connect to your inner satisfaction pathways, then happiness, health and longevity are all measurably improved. People reported to Gallup Polls that when they are able to work in a fashion that is based on their strengths, they are three times more likely to report an excellent quality of life and six times more likely to be engaged with their work. Montessori schools, monasteries and places where people "consider their work as a calling rather than a job" are virtually devoid of burnout [4].

So how can one find a way to work and live that they're engaged with, while avoiding the perils of burnout as described above? We don't claim to have the single magical answer but hope this chapter will provide some useful strategies with which to approach the challenge we all face.

Burnout

Physician burnout has been described as both a public health crisis and an epidemic. It is rising in prevalence among all physicians, and has been found to exist at a very high level specifically among urologists, as illustrated by recent data suggesting nearly 40% of urologists are currently meeting burnout criteria [5]. First described by Dr. Herbert Freudenberger in his 1980 book Burn Out: The High Cost of High Achievement, a person with burn-out is "overcome by fatigue and frustration which are usually brought about when a job, a cause, a way of life, or relationship fails to produce the expected reward" [6]. Furthermore, those who suffer burn out are usually high achievers.

While burnout among physicians is a relatively new phenomenon, it has exploded into awareness and is accurately described as a public health crisis. A 2019 report published by the Harvard T. H. Chan School of Public Health, the Harvard Global Health Institute, the Massachusetts Medical Society and Massachusetts Health and Hospital Association suggests the origin of this crisis can be in part traced to the 1999 publication of the Institute of Medicine's "To Err is Human" report, which ushered in a new era of medicine with a newly heightened regulatory focus on physician practice, quality, and accountability [7]. This new direction went on to create a field dominated by "rewards, punishments, and pay for performance." Burnout stems from the disconnection between the noble and caring profession that physicians thought they were signing up for, and the content of their day-to-day practice.

The consequence of this attention to all-new ways of trying to herd physicians towards "better" practice has been a significant loss of autonomy and the addition of new extrinsic demands, mostly for documentation of various sorts. The great majority of these new stresses are enacted through the bane of contemporary practice: the electronic medical record.

Frustrations are integral to life and work, but frustrations that exist beyond our control, such as those that may come from disconnected management or corporate failure, may lead to deep unhappiness. Fully expressed, this sacrifice of control can be similar to "learned helplessness" (LH), a biologic model of the interface between control, the inability to exert control, and depression. LH has been shown to create 8 of the 9 criteria for depression as expressed in the DSM9, where just 5 are required to meet the diagnosis of clinical depression [8]. Thus, inability to exert control when severe or important enough can lead to elements of depression and is a key component of burnout.

Change is necessary. Retaking control is necessary. While there are individual skills and methods that one can employ to minimize the negative effects of this loss of autonomy and increase in administrative and electronic medical record (EMR)-base demand, laying the responsibility for burnout management at the feet of the practitioners has been aptly compared to telling drivers to wear seatbelts instead of repairing dangerous roads and broken stoplights [7]. We break strategies preventing/combating this crisis into two categories:

1. Things you cannot change alone (but should strongly advocate for) = Systemic Change.
2. Things that you can change about yourself and about your work = Self Change.

Systemic Strategies

It is said that every system is perfectly designed to get the results that it gets. We seem to have a system that is designed to burn out 50% of its workforce. In a response to this, the Massachusetts/Harvard report makes three initial recommendations, all of which address system-level deficiencies:

1. Aggressive availability and integration of physician help services into the practice environment.
2. EMR reform/changes in how billing, documentation and the interface between patient care and documentation occurs

3. Institutional-level creation of a Chief Wellness Officer: a person responsible for the health and wellness of the physicians at each institution.

To achieve these changes, physicians must be actively engaged and participatory. You have to advocate on your own behalf. If there is a meeting about physician wellness, go to it. If there is a ballot regarding the Chief Wellness Officer, cast your vote. If there are physician help services available to you, learn how to access them when needed. As an individual physician at a large institution, it can be easy to have a learned helplessness attitude towards system changes, but that is an attitude that champions the status quo.

Self Strategies

While we feel that active engagement and support of the systemic changes outlined above by all physicians are both critical to the change we need, there are things you yourself can do to prevent and combat burnout. We further subdivide these into those that are specifically job related and those that are not-just-job-related.

EMR Management:

We expect that virtually all readers will recognize the demands made on our practice by electronic documentation and administrative tasks. In a study published in 2018, electronic documentation tasks and burnout are closely related and this relationship likely surprises no practitioner [9]. A separate survey in the *Journal of the American Medical Association* identified the EMR as physician's number one "pain point", and in some settings physicians spend literally twice as much time interfacing with their EMR and documentation needs as they do with patients [10, 11]. This is flatly not why any of us went to medical school. However, In addition to supporting and encouraging the systemic change that is needed in this domain, an individual can also work to optimize their individual interface with their EMR. Aggressive effort to become a high-level user will pay off over time. Can you afford to take a full day off to deepen your knowledge and facility with the EMR? Yes. Think about the pay off in terms of a career's worth of earlier departure from the office, fewer hours at home charting, and generally faster and more efficient interfaces with patients.

To the point of EMR usage, a scribe can (we hear) be a life-changing addition to one's practice. A scribe is a data entry specialist whose sole purpose is to interface with the EMR in real-time during patient visits and the data supporting their use is promising. A prospective study of over 25,000 emergency department visits found that visits per hour, relative value unit (RVU) production and patient satisfaction were all significantly improved with the addition of a scribe [12]. A meta-analysis of five studies also showed improvements in clinician satisfaction, productivity, time-related efficiencies, revenue, and patient-clinician interactions in multiple types of physician settings [13]. A 2010 study on the usage of scribes in a urology office showed a dramatic improvement in physician satisfaction with office hours, improving from 19 to 69% with the usage of a scribe [14].

Job-Fit:

In her book, *The Happiness Project*, Gretchen Rubin writes, "People who love their work bring an intensity and enthusiasm that is impossible to match through sheer diligence" [15]. Studies show that physicians who spend at least 20% of their professional effort on the type of work they find the most meaningful are at significantly lower risk for burnout [16]. Similarly, Mark Mason proposes a strategy: "choose the struggle you love." If one accepts that success in any endeavor will require a long and sustained struggle, then shouldn't one choose the struggle that resonates the most with them? In *Fit Matters: How to Love Your Job*, authors Carrick and Dunaway argue that when you combine rigorous self-knowledge with an understanding of an organization's culture, then you have the tools to make career decisions that will lead to better job satisfaction and improved performance [17]. They illustrate 6 elements of Work Fit: job fit, culture fit, relationship fit, lifestyle fit, and financial fit.

For the young urologist, this may provide some degree of guidance with career selection. Would you be happiest in the operating room until late at night perfecting your outcomes? Do you prefer teaching residents over laboratory work? Are you happier organizing the system that you work in than when confronted with a huge stack of patients to see in a day? They all require work, and you didn't sign up for medical school to avoid work, but they are different and can represent very different sets of challenges. Chose the challenge that will be the most gratifying to you.

A critical aspect of work-life synergy is the culture of the organization you choose to place yourself within. As much as strength-based leadership can guide you new successes, toxic management can surely crush happiness and your soul. Quoting an excellent Mayo Clinic paper on the responsibility of management to prevent burnout: "Mistakenly, most hospitals, medical centers, and practice groups operate under the framework that burnout and professional satisfaction are solely the responsibility of the individual physician. This frequently results in organizations pursuing a narrow list of "solutions" that are unlikely to result in meaningful progress (eg, stress management work-shops and individual training in mindfulness/resilience). Such strategies neglect the organizational factors that are the primary drivers of physician burnout and are correctly viewed with skepticism by physicians as an insincere effort by the organization to address the problem. Casting the issue as a personal problem can also lead individual physicians to pursue solutions that are personally beneficial but detrimental to the organization and society, such as reducing professional work effort or pursuing a concierge practice model" [3, 10]

Paradoxically, as a critical-shortage specialty, urologists are in a strong place to drive that conversation, and to encourage change as we've discussed. We strongly recommend that not only do all leadership-bound physicians read them carefully, but also new graduates will benefit from understanding and identification of the markers of good work culture.

Self-Reflection/Self-Direction:

Are you happy? How can you get happier? If you're reading this book, we assume you've been successful in school, so can you simply apply the principles that got you through college? Is it as simple as just going out and earning more money? A highly cited paper from the psychological world assesses the measures of success in terms of objective (status, pay) as compared to subjective measures such as satisfaction, and found that not only are the two poorly related, but higher status/pay had no relationship on job satisfaction. Even more interesting was the fact that there did appear to be a relationship that functioned in the opposite direction—higher satisfaction with one's job resulted in higher pay/status [18].

What has been shown to generate happiness? If we are to go down the analytic rabbit-hole towards the creation of happiness, we will find that there in fact are a few good answers. Each individual will have a different framework, but the key is to thoughtfully generate this framework. We submit that the step of writing a personal, and/or family mission statement can be a key step. Experts in this field suggest one that is focused more on principles and "things I/we believe", than on tangible goals. Subsequent issues, challenges, questions and opportunities can then be considered in the context of an individualized framework of values and principles [19, 20].

When you are formulating your manifesto, it can be helpful to consider what Ethan Roland has identified as the eight different "capitals" that compose real wealth: financial and material capital; living capital which refers to the health of your environment; social capital, or the connections we have with friends and family; experiential capital which is gained through experiences; intellectual capital, which is found through knowledge and ideas; spiritual capital; cultural capital, which can only be held by a group of people; and finally, health and well-being capital [21]. When you consider your personal wealth and happiness, consider each of these and that fact that, like the stock market, they are dynamic and can be added to or depleted. Using these categories with your own values assigned to each will help you to craft the manifesto.

One domain that deserves specific discussion is the concept of money. Quite likely no topic related to work, or the discussion surrounding a job, gets more time than that of the compensation. This implicit value permeates current culture: from professional athletes who seem to want no more than to have the highest possible contract, to endless water cooler discussions about recruitment opportunities and what someone heard was being paid in a different venue, we appear to value nothing more than income, and use income as a profoundly important measure of the quality of a job. And yet, the social science underlying this is fairly clear: humans greatly over-value the anticipated future happiness associated with more money. Psychologists refer to this phenomenon as affective forecasting, and the short story is that we are all quite poor at it. Examples abound that are worth considering: removing an hourlong commute can make you as much happier as making an additional $40,000 per year. Additionally, people that live in areas where happiness is high will adapt to that local level of happiness (or unhappiness). And when one studies the impact of abrupt cash infusion, in the form of a lottery win, one sees how more money quite often doesn't make things better and can in fact make things much worse. We'll leave it to you to work out how your personal affective forecasting may be mis-valuing things that you are working towards, but we strongly suggest that you critically evaluate your concepts of how much happiness you ascribe to future money, and especially in the context of the other values in your life such as family, social interaction, experiences (such as travel and vacation). While it is true that scheduling these diversions is easier with more money, there clearly is a point beyond which one's focus is off the mark. Excellent discussions of this specific topic, and happiness broadly, are available in Laurie Santos' "Happiness Lab" podcast, and directly related to surgery/ urology in "Operating with Zen" moderated by Phil Pierorazio, MD, among others.

Think Differently

Consider work-life balance. This construct suggests that we must constantly take from one to give to the other to achieve the balanced end. If we re-frame this concept as work-life harmony, suddenly we can consider the that work and non-work may mutually co-exist, one complementing the other, harmoniously. This is an example of thinking differently. Thinking differently is a powerful weapon against the enemy, burnout. An excellent, and brief, book, *7 Ways to Think Differently*, by Looby MacNamara is a great starting point to begin doing just that [22]. The 7 ways of thinking differently can be used to approach personal, social, and global issues; from figuring out how your schedule will accommodate a trip to the dentist to how your healthcare system can optimize physician productivity without sacrificing well-being.

The authors propose seven categories: Abundance thinking, solutions thinking, systems thinking, thinking like nature, cooperative thinking, thinking for the future, and from thinking to doing. We believe that benefit may be found by focusing on the first three. Abundance thinking, as opposed to scarcity thinking, starts from the basic assumption that there is enough. There is enough for you individually, for society currently, and for society in the future. In this competitive health care market, it is easy to worry about the urology group across the street making more money, getting more cases, or increasing their market share. This is scarcity thinking which is driven by fear. Beginning with the basic assumption that there are plenty of cases to go around, one has the room to apply your focus to things like how to do the best job, provide the best care, how to create a workplace that is enjoyable for everyone. Abundance thinking allows you to shift from quantity to quality, scarcity of resources to flow or resources, and potentially from priority emphasis on financial wealth to a broader construct of wealth.

Solutions thinking begins with the basic assumption that for any given problem, there is a solution. When faced with the bureaucracy of medicine, it can be very easy to fall into he learned helpless mode that was described earlier in this chapter. Solutions thinking jumps past that by assuming that a solution exists, we just have to find our way to it. This is a far more empowering starting point from which to approach challenges, and it generates creativity rather than passivity. Rather than being reactive, you can be proactive. To adopt corporate jargon, challenges become opportunities. The deepest lesson from 50 years of learned helplessness data is that the default position of humans when confronted by stressors is passivity; it is the secondary application of control/ avoidance behavior that prevents anxiety and depression from occurring. Solve, don't suffer!

Finally, systems thinking requires a shift from contemplating individual parts to thinking about wholes, a move from thinking about components to the relationships between the things that are made of those components, the proverbial forest for the trees. Your clinic is a system, possibly inside a hospital system, which may be part of a larger healthcare system. Like a Russian nesting doll, each one is whole in itself and held within another whole. Fundamental to systems thinking is that small changes can have rippling effects. Accordingly, your small actions can have meaningful and significant consequences. Because those effects are often not predictable, it is important to be responsive to what emerges. Systems thinking can be an empowering way to approach what may otherwise seem like a Sisyphean task. And at the core of these useful thought exercises is the imperative to work for solutions, both small and large.

Self-Care: Eat, Move, Learn

Eat: We should all be eating better. As we routinely tell our patients, what we put into our bodies has consequences. Whether it be adequate fluids and citrate to counteract stone formation or less cigarettes to decrease bladder cancer, what goes in makes a difference. As Dan Buettner, author of the much-recommended "Blue Zones" books that examine the characteristics of the longest-living communities on earth puts it: "The calculus of aging offers us two options: We can live a shorter life with more years of disability, or we can live the longest possible life with the fewest bad years. As my centenarian friends showed me, the choice is largely up to us."

Dietary contemplation is beyond the scope of this chapter, but were we to suggest books for friends, colleagues or thoughtful patients we would include Buettner's book as well as Michael Pollan's *Food Rules: An Eater's Manual* F [23]. Quoting Pollan: "Eat real food, not too much, mostly vegetables".

Move: One core of our happiness is an intact and well-functioning physical being. Recently, attention and concern have been directed towards surgery itself, and within urology laparoscopic surgery especially has been cited as a potential cause of physical and musculoskeletal injury. One recent article suggested an "impending epidemic" of injury from modern surgical volumes and techniques [24]. Fortunately, a large recent survey found no relationship found to surgical type, gender, volume or duration of practice, despite the fact that half of those with pain blamed it on their surgical ergonomics. So, work on! While this is certainly an encouraging finding, the same study refocused attention on the importance of self-care: exercise and BMI were related to rates of back pain, with lower BMIs and higher rates of exercise both appearing protective.

And how can one achieve those lower BMIs? Imagine, for a moment, that there was a drug that was available to you (and your patients!) that had the following properties:

- It made you smarter.
- It made you happier.
- It made you 20–30% less likely to die at a given point.
- It made you stronger and faster.
- It was preventative of hip fracture and bone density loss.
- It prevented depression as well as hypertension.
- It prevented kidney stones and improved voiding function.

Would you take it? Would you prescribe it? What if it was free? Well, it is, and we call it "exercise". So there. And while commonly available, the routine swallowing of the exercise pill can be quite a challenge. It turns out that, despite being truly a wonder drug, not everyone likes to take it. But they should [25].

Learn: After 4 years of college, 4 years of medical school, 5 or 6 years of residency, and anywhere from 1–3 years of fellowship, it is understandable to feel as if you have finally "finished" your education. However, while all of this training has helped you become an outstanding Urologist, it may not have given you all the skills you need to be a Medical Director, Informatics Office, Chief Wellness Officer, or Associate Dean. Explore the opportunities available for professional development at your institution, outside institutions, or through professional societies such as the American College of Surgeons, or the American Association of Medical Colleges. Mastering new skill sets leads to self-efficacy and self-efficacy is antithetical to burnout.

Purchase Time

The two currencies that can be used in exchange for happiness are, in varying ratios, money and time. Can you generate more of one with the other? Time surely can be spent generating money—for more on that topic, refer to that modern concept "work". More interestingly, money can also be spent generating time, and yet we do bad internal math on this strategy. A large study spanning multiple countries showed that the usage of time-saving strategies, with a cost, had the benefit of improved happiness as well as relief of time-stress [26]. The findings in this study held across income levels and across societies, underscoring the durability of the concept. To quote the authors: "...people who spend money on time-saving purchases report greater life satisfaction".

The study itself focused on the completion of "unenjoyable daily tasks"; beyond that there were no specifics and we would leave the identification of exactly what that means to each reader. Grocery shopping? Consider a service that delivers groceries or even pre-made food to your home, many are available. Mowing the lawn? Hire the neighbor's kid or a service. Housecleaning? Maid. Reframe your thinking not to consider these services as luxuries, but rather buying back your valuable time. Certainly, many readers will observe that they find great solace and peace in gardening, cleaning, et cetera. The arithmetic will be different for everyone.

Conclusion

Wellness is important, but it is not easy. It requires thought, attention, and ongoing work throughout your career. Seize control! What happiness, and wellness, look like will be different for everyone. We hope that this chapter has provided some jumping off points for exploring what a happy and successful career as a urologist will look like for you.

Key Points

- Create Happiness

    i. Write your individual and/or family mission statement. Focus on principles and values, not as much goals. Review periodically e.g. every New Years.
    ii. Consider using your money to purchase experiences and more time

- Assess whether you're burned out. Take the MBI, 5 mins: available here through the National Academy of Medicine website, https://nam.edu/valid-reliable-survey-instruments-measure-burnout-well-work-related-dimensions/
- Control your career and turn it to your desires. Make it a vehicle for your happiness.
- Encourage your institution to install a Chief Wellness Officer.
- Engage and develop an EMR management strategy. Consider a scribe. Engage your EMR vendor to help make it easier for you. Support change and advancement.
- Optimize your time and include validated devices:

    i. Exercise. Find a way, find something fun to do. It doesn't have to be hard, just but it does have to be enjoyable so that you'll keep doing it.
    ii. Eat Well
    iii. Meditate
    iv. Sing. Especially in groups. It lowers stress, relieves anxiety, and decreases cortisol levels [27]
    v. Actively work to develop and maintain relationships with friends and family
    vi. Build community.

- Great resource for all things burnout and happiness-related:

    i. http://www.ucdenver.edu/academics/colleges/medicalschool/facultyAffairs/Resilience/Documents/BurnoutPreventionMatrix-V4.3.pdf
    ii. Podcasts: https://www.happinesslab.fm and https://podcasts.apple.com/us/podcast/operate-with-zen/id1579495428 (available on all major podcast systems).
    iii. Stanford's Well MD Materials, www.wellmd.stanford.edu
    iv. AMA Steps Forward Program, www.Stepsforward.org

v. AAMC Leadership Development, https://www.aamc.org/members/leadership

vi. ACGME Well-Being Initiatives, https://www.acgme.org/What-We-Do/Initiatives/Physician-Well-Being

vii. American College of Physicians Well-Being Resources, https://www.acponline.org/practice-resources/physician-well-being-and-professional-satisfaction

viii. National Academy of Medicine Clinician Well-Being Knowledge Hub.

ix. https://www.nam.edu/clinicianwellbeing/

x. www.oneactofkindness.org

xi. www.gretchenrubin.com/

xii. www.thehappymd.com/.

References

1. Simonton DK. Greatness: Who Makes History and Why: The Guilford Press; 1994
2. Maslach C. Burnout : the cost of caring. Cambridge, MA: Malor Books; 2003. p. xxiv, 276.
3. Shanafelt TD, Noseworthy JH. Executive Leadership and Physician Well-being: Nine Organizational Strategies to Promote Engagement and Reduce Burnout. Mayo Clin Proc. 2017;92(1):129–46. https://doi.org/10.1016/j.mayocp.2016.10.004 PubMed PMID: 27871627.
4. Farber BA, Cherniss K. Stress and burnout in the human service professions: Elsevier; 1983. 272 p.
5. Amanda C, North PHM, Fang R, Sener A, McNeil BK, Franc-Guimond J, Meeks WD, Schlossberg SM, Gonzalez C, Quentin J, Clemens. Burnout in Urology: findings from the AUA Annual Census. Urol Pract. 2016;2018(5):489–94.
6. Freudenberger HJ, Richelson G. Burn-out : the high cost of high achievement, 1st ed. Garden City, N.Y.: Anchor Press; 1980. xxii, 214 p.
7. Ashish K Jha ARI, Alain A Chaoui, Steven Defossez, Maryanne C Bombaugh, Yael R Miller. A Crisis in Health Care: A Call to Action on Physician Burnout. In: Massachusetts Medical Society MHaHA, Harvard T. H. Chan School of Public Health, and Harvard Global Health Institute, editor. Massachusetts Medical Society; 2019.
8. Maier SF, Seligman ME. Learned helplessness at fifty: Insights from neuroscience. Psychol Rev. 2016;123(4):349–67. https://doi.org/10.1037/rev0000033.PubMedPMID:27337390; PubMedCentralPMCID:PMCPMC4920136.
9. Gardner RL, Cooper E, Haskell J, Harris DA, Poplau S, Kroth PJ, et al. Physician stress and burnout: the impact of health information technology. J Am Med Inform Assoc. 2019;26 (2):106–14. https://doi.org/10.1093/jamia/ocy145 PubMed PMID: 30517663.
10. Shanafelt TD, Dyrbye LN, West CP. Addressing Physician Burnout: The Way Forward. JAMA. 2017;317(9):901–2. https://doi.org/10.1001/jama.2017.0076 PubMed PMID: 28196201.
11. Rotenstein LS, Torre M, Ramos MA, Rosales RC, Guille C, Sen S, et al. Prevalence of burnout among physicians: a systematic review. JAMA. 2018;320(11):1131–50. https://doi.org/10.1001/jama.2018.12777.PubMedPMID:30326495;PubMedCentralPMCID: PMCPMC6233645.
12. Shuaib W, Hilmi J, Caballero J, Rashid I, Stanazai H, Ajanovic A, et al. Impact of a scribe program on patient throughput, physician productivity, and patient satisfaction in a

community-based emergency department. Health Inf J. 2017:1460458217692930. Epub 2017/03/01. https://doi.org/10.1177/1460458217692930. PubMed PMID: 29239230.

13. Shultz CG, Holmstrom HL. The use of medical scribes in health care settings: a systematic review and future directions. J Am Board Fam Med. 2015;28(3):371–81. https://doi.org/10.3122/jabfm.2015.03.140224 PubMed PMID: 25957370.

14. Koshy S, Feustel PJ, Hong M, Kogan BA. Scribes in an ambulatory urology practice: patient and physician satisfaction. J Urol. 2010;184(1):258–62. https://doi.org/10.1016/j.juro.2010.03.040 PubMed PMID: 20483153.

15. Rubin G. The happiness project : or why I spent a year trying to sing in the morning, clean my closets, fight right, read Aristotle, and generally have more fun, 1st ed. New York, NY: Harper; 2009. xiv, 301 p. p.

16. Shanafelt TD, West CP, Sloan JA, Novotny PJ, Poland GA, Menaker R, et al. Career fit and burnout among academic faculty. Arch Intern Med. 2009;169(10):990–5. https://doi.org/10.1001/archinternmed.2009.70 PubMed PMID: 19468093.

17. Moe Carrick CD. Fit Matters. Palmyra, VA: Maven House Press; 2017.

18. Abele AE, Spurk D. How do objective and subjective career success interrelate over time? J Occup Organ Psychol. 2009;82:803–24. https://doi.org/10.1348/096317909X470924.

19. Feiler B. Want to Give Your Family Value and Purpose: Write a Mission Statement. The Atlantic. 2013;25:2013.

20. Parker-Pope T. Creating a New Mission Statement. NY Times. 2015;5:2015.

21. Rowland E. Eight Forms of Capital. Permaculture. 2011.

22. MacNamara L. 7 Ways to Think Differently. Hampshire, United Kingdom: Permanent Publications; 2014.

23. Pollan M. Food rules : an eater's manual. New York: Penguin Books; 2009. xx, 140 p. p.

24. Park A, Lee G, Seagull FJ, Meenaghan N, Dexter D. Patients benefit while surgeons suffer: an impending epidemic. J Am Coll Surg. 2010;210(3):306–13. https://doi.org/10.1016/j.jamcollsurg.2009.10.017 PubMed PMID: 20193893.

25. Fletcher GF, Landolfo C, Niebauer J, Ozemek C, Arena R, Lavie CJ. Reprint of: Promoting Physical Activity and Exercise: JACC Health Promotion Series. J Am Coll Cardiol. 2018;72 (23 Pt B):3053–70. https://doi.org/10.1016/j.jacc.2018.10.025. PubMed PMID: 30522636.

26. Whillans AV, Dunn EW, Smeets P, Bekkers R, Norton MI. Buying time promotes happiness. Proc Natl Acad Sci USA. 2017;114(32):8523–7. Epub 2017/07/24. https://doi.org/10.1073/pnas.1706541114. PubMed PMID: 28739889; PubMed Central PMCID: PMCPMC5559044.

27. Horn S. Imperfect harmony: finding happiness singing with others, 1st edn. Algonquin Books of Chapel Hill; 2013, 284 p.

Chapter 18
The Power of History and Leveraging Past Institutional Success

Sutchin R. Patel

Why is History Important?

When I have been asked "Why is studying history important?" three famous quotations come to mind:

Those who do not remember the past are condemned to repeat it.—George Santayana

If I have seen further, it is by standing on the shoulders of giants.—Isaac Newton

It is not the strongest of the species that survives but the most adaptable.—Charles Darwin

Understanding our history can help us learn from the mistakes of the past, it can help us to advance our current knowledge by building upon past experiences, and most importantly it can allow us to adapt to the inevitable changes that will occur throughout our careers.

In the case of the COVID-19 pandemic, history has played an important role in helping construct our response of how to combat the pandemic. An understanding of the 1918 H1N1 pandemic helped us to realize the benefit of many non-pharmaceutical measures such as the use of quarantine, restrictions on public gatherings, the use of face masks, and hand washing/hygiene [1]. Mask wearing is not a new phenomenon when it comes to protecting ourselves, as people have used masks for hundreds of years in an early, though not completely understood, attempt to halt the spread of disease. By building upon our historical understanding of facemasks and further exploring the importance of filtration efficiency as well as mask fit and placement, the use of facial coverings has been a simple but powerful tool in helping us combat our current pandemic [2]. Social distancing has been cited as one of the pillars to help prevent the spread of COVID-19 and there have been

S. R. Patel (✉)
Department of Urology, University of Wisconsin School of Medicine and Public Health, Madison, WI 53705, USA
e-mail: sutchin_patel@yahoo.com

© The Author(s), under exclusive license to Springer Nature Switzerland AG 2022
S. Y. Nakada and S. R. Patel (eds.), *Navigating Organized Urology*,
https://doi.org/10.1007/978-3-031-05540-9_18

numerous historical studies that have illustrated the spread of aerosolized pathogens [3]. It was during the SARS epidemic in 2002 that authorities set the aerosolized at-risk distance as 6 feet. In one case, a man with SARS on a three-hour flight from Hong Kong to Beijing infected twenty-two people, five of whom died. Of the twenty-three passengers in the same row or up to three rows in front of the index patient, eight fell ill, however people seven rows away (approximately 18 feet away) developed SARS too. It has thus been recognized that depending on factors such as temperature, humidity, air circulation, and coughing or sneezing, aerosolized droplets can be propelled more than twenty feet [3]. However, whenever we turn to history to extract lessons that can be applied to a current problem it is important to examine the past events through the social, political, and scientific lens of its own time and to not fall into the trap of focusing solely on similarities but to also understand key differences in the events [4]. During the frightening times of plagues and pandemics the greatest gift that history can give us is perspective and hope. Hope, that like our resilient ancestors, we too will endure and survive our current turbulent times.

Teaching the History of Urology

A survey of urology residency program directors in the United States found that 83% of respondents felt that the history of urology should be taught in residency [5]. When asked why they believed it should be taught, 97% felt that it provided residents with a sense of historical perspective and connection to the past, 49% stated that it could provide better judgment and reasoning, 64% believed it could provide a more critical approach to contemporary surgery and 66% felt it could lead to a deeper understanding of professionalism. Although urologic history could bridge many aspects of resident education, in terms of the United States Accreditation Council for Graduate Medical Education (ACGME) core competencies, it would likely best fit under professionalism, and there is a growing literature that shows that history can also be used to help teach ethics [6–8].

In 1902, Sir William Osler stated that the history of medicine could be taught "by lectures, historical clubs, questioning students during rounds as well as informally over 'beer and baccy' (tobacco)." However, Osler lamented that, "in the present crowded state of the curriculum it does not seem desirable to add the History of Medicine as a compulsory subject" [9]. The increased time constraints on formal teaching during residency can make it difficult to teach the history of urology. These same time constraints in a hectic medical school curriculum were found to be the primary cause for a decline in medical history instruction by Genevieve Miller, a medical historian. She would write "Antiquarianism and mediocre teaching have tended to retard medical history in American medical education… most medical educators today are unaware of its positive values. Only by being relevant and excellently presented will the subject be accepted as an essential part of the training of physicians" [10].

The history of urology, when taught in residency, has to be relevant and is best incorporated into what we do on a regular basis. It can be taught on rounds or in the operating room. A personal example was that while on my pediatric urology rotation as a resident, the use of the Denis Browne retractor led my attending, Dr. Caldamone, to ask the simple question "Who was Denis Browne?" This ultimately led to a history paper on Browne's contributions to pediatric urology [11]. Curiosity can be a great tool to help teach history—ask Why do we do what we do today? How did we do it in the past? Who are some of the eponymous names for surgical procedures, instruments, diseases, or anatomical structures? Writing a history paper can also be a great project for medical students interested in urology as it generally does not require the significant time needed for an independent research project and it serves as a great introduction to our field.

Besides incorporating the history of urology into rounds and the operating room, it can also be taught as introductory slides to grand rounds presentations, in a journal club setting (reviewing seminal papers in our field) and in some cases as dedicated lectures (generally covering important large topics in our field, for example, the history of the development of the cystoscope, the history and evolution of the treatment of prostate cancer, etc.). Of the urology residency program directors queried in a 2013 survey, when asked how the history of urology should be taught in residency: 66% stated that it should be taught on rounds or in the operating room as well as introductory slides to presentation, 64% felt it should be taught in a journal club setting and 49% believed it should be taught in formal history lectures [5].

What resources do we have to help teach the history of urology? There are a few texts available that are solely devoted to the history of urology however none of them are comprehensive and many of them do not include the more current history of our field [12–15]. A few more modern but field-specific historical texts include "Urolithiasis: A Comprehensive History" and "The History of Technologic Advancements in Urology" [16, 17].

Journal articles provide an easily accessible and fresh source of historical perspective. Hugh Hampton Young in the foreward of the 1st issue of *The Journal of Urology* stated "It is therefore evident that some common meeting place is extremely desirable—some medium in which all types of papers upon the field of common interest may appear—archives of Urology—historical, embryological, anatomical, biochemical, pharmacological, pathological, bacteriological, surgical and medical, experimental and clinical" [18]. In 1973, *Urology* (Gold Journal) was founded and in its first issue, Pablo Morales, the journal's founding editor, wrote that "The success of the journal will depend not only on its appeal to the authors… but also to the audience that reads most of what is published" further stating that "other features will include essays on the history of urology" [19]. However, since 2009 *The Journal of Urology* and *Urology* have taken a divergent approach to publishing history manuscripts with *The Journal of Urology* no longer publishing them and Urology having thus seen an increase in published history articles (35 articles from 2009 to 2017) [20]. A number of other urology journals do publish history articles including *The Canadian Journal of Urology, Journal of*

Endourology and the *Journal of Pediatric Urology*. The *International Journal of Urologic History*, debuted in 2021, and under Dr. John Philips as editor is a journal solely dedicated to publishing urologic history articles. Given the ease of performing a literature search, for many, PubMed can be a great starting point to learn more about a urology history topic. Another good source for urology history are the annual volumes of *de Historia Urologiae Europaeae* published by the History Office of the European Association of Urology.

The William P. Didusch Center of Urologic History

We are fortunate that our specialty has its own dedicated museum and one that has been well organized and curated over the years. The story of our museum starts with William P. Didusch, who began his career as the staff artist for the then newly created Brady Urological Institute under Hugh Hampton Young and would spend his entire life illustrating and thus helping teach urology to many future generations of urologists (Fig. 18.1).

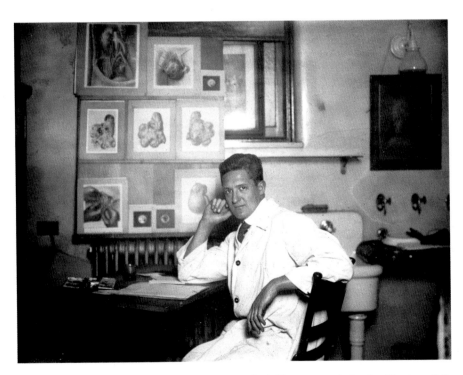

Fig. 18.1 William P. Didusch (1895–1981). Medical illustrator and the 1st Curator of the William P. Didusch Urological Museum, as it was called at the time [*Courtesy of the William P. Didusch Center for Urologic History*]

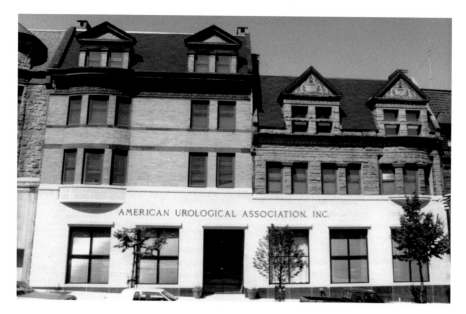

Fig. 18.2 The Original Headquarters of the AUA (1120 North Charles Street, Baltimore MD) [*Courtesy of the William P. Didusch Center for Urologic History*]

William P. Didusch studied from 1913 to 1915 under Max Brödel, the famous medical illustrator, who founded the Department of Art as Applied to Medicine at the Johns Hopkins School of Medicine, the first full-fledged department of medical art established by a medical institution [21]. In 1915 Brödel offered Didusch the opportunity to become the staff artist for the newly created Brady Urological Institute at the Johns Hopkins Hospital under Hugh Hampton Young. In 1949 he was appointed an instructor in urology at the Johns Hopkins Hospital by Dr William W. Scott and in 1953 he became the Executive Secretary of the AUA. From 1928 to 1967 he served as the director of exhibits for the annual convention of the AUA. He was prolific in his work, serving as art editor for *The Journal of Urology*, illustrating 18 medical texts starting with Young's Practice of Urology (1926), and creating illustrations in over 600 medical articles. In 1968, Didusch proposed the creation of a urologic museum and donated his collection of drawings to the AUA for that purpose. In 1971 the American Urologic Association established the William P. Didusch Urological Museum at the Association's Headquarters in Baltimore (1120 North Charles Street, Baltimore MD) and appointed William Didusch as its first curator [22] (Fig. 18.2). The museum's initial collection began with Didusch's vast collection of urological drawings as well as a few instruments. Since then the collection has grown significantly and the museum was moved to the new AUA Headquarters in Linthicum, MD in October 1989 (Fig. 18.3).

With the museum residing at the AUA Headquarters in Linthicum, MD, I would encourage any urologist visiting the headquarters or the city of Baltimore as well as anyone interested in the history of urology to consider a stop at the museum. Letting

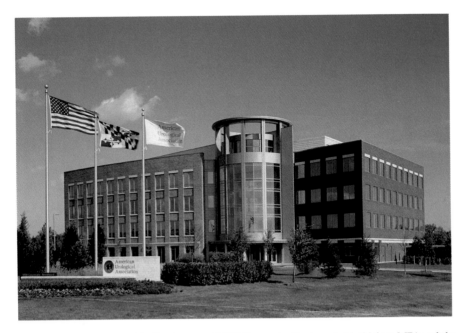

Fig. 18.3 The Current AUA Headquarters (1000 Corporate Boulevard, Linthicium MD) and the site of the William P. Didusch Center of Urologic History [*Courtesy of the William P. Didusch Center for Urologic History*]

the museum staff know in advance of your visit may allow you to get a private tour of the museum, including its collection of cystoscopes and urologic texts (Figs. 18.4 and 18.5). The museum also houses the history exhibit from that year's annual AUA meeting for a portion of the year. The museum and its staff can be a great resource for questions about the history of urology or for any historical research in our field or about the AUA. The current website for the museum is www.urologichistory.museum.

History as a Source of Institutional Pride

> I like to see a man proud of the place in which he lives. I like to see a man live so that his place will be proud of him.—Abraham Lincoln

When we are taught American History throughout grade school and in high school, it gives us a sense of civic pride and further binds us together as a country. It allows us to connect to our past and feel that we are a part of something much greater. In this same way, teaching institutional history can foster a greater connection among members of an academic department and lead to institutional pride.

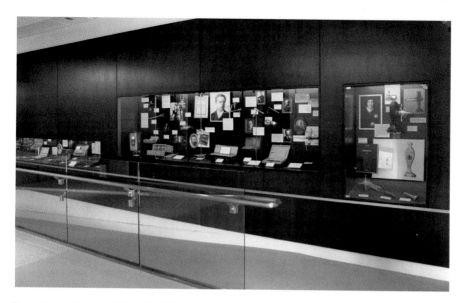

Fig. 18.4 Inside the William P. Didusch Museum—The Development of the Cystoscope Exhibit. [*Courtesy of the William P. Didusch Center for Urologic History*]

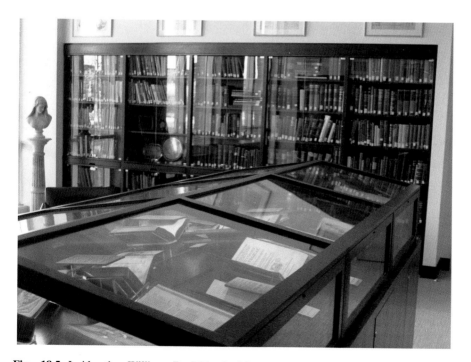

Fig. 18.5 Inside the William P. Didusch Museum—Library Room [*Courtesy of the William P. Didusch Center for Urologic History*]

The history of a department should help the current residents and faculty feel connected to the accomplishments of the past and to further connect them to their mentors. An understanding of institutional history helps us map how a department started, what changes it underwent and what those that came before us accomplished thus leading us to better and more importantly predict where it is going. Many departments have a hall or a room with pictures of past graduating classes or portraits of former department chairs. But how many residents or even faculty members know something about the faces in the pictures? These can be a great starting point for teaching institutional history.

Appreciating past institutional success can also be used to inspire future accomplishments. An important part of this is recognizing and celebrating current success. When a nation wins a medal at the Olympics the success of that individual is celebrated by the entire nation. The same can apply to academic departments. The success of an individual within a department can lead to institutional pride and further inspire others in the department. Furthermore, the recognition the individual receives sends the message that his/her work and success is valued. Do not underestimate these shared experiences and the positive effect it can have on departmental morale.

Another vehicle to both chronicle and formally acknowledge the accomplishments of individuals in a department is a departmental newsletter, or regular communication. Starting one does not always take a significant time commitment, but does require careful review for content and influence. The newsletter can be used to acknowledge the achievements/work/awards of individuals, announce upcoming lectureships, introduce new residents, faculty and staff members, and serve as a record of the history of the department. Each newsletter is a snapshot of the department at the time and the combined archive of newsletters can chronicle the history of the department. Other advantages to a newsletter are that it can be sent to former alumni to keep them in touch with the institution and can also be used to help in departmental philanthropy.

History for the Private Practice Urologist

The institutional history of hospitals and physician practices in your area can be helpful in navigating local changes in health care. This historical perspective can be difficult when first joining a new practice but speaking to those that have been practicing in your region for some time can be helpful in understanding how hospital systems have developed and possibly underlying politics in the region. Like any history, understanding the past may help to prepare for future changes in health care in your particular region.

Anecdotally, I have also found that patients may enjoy learning the history of urology. Whether it be how catheters were developed or the development and evolution of how we treat urologic disease today, a comment on the relevant urologic history regarding a patient's condition can many times lead to an

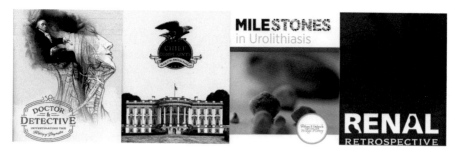

Fig. 18.6   Annual AUA History Exhibit Publications [*Courtesy of the William P. Didusch Center for Urologic History*]

interesting conversation. Each year the William P. Didusch Center for Urologic History puts together a history exhibit in the exhibit hall of the annual meeting. At the exhibit each year is a free publication outlining the current exhibit and short vignettes on medical and urologic history (Fig. 18.6). I have found these publications to make for great reading material in the waiting room of our office as a number of patients have commented on how much they enjoyed reading them.

Professor Emeritus

The title "Professor Emeritus" used to be given to select professors after their mandatory retirement age of 65. Emeritus in Latin means "deserved" or "earned" and with the abolishment of mandatory retirement for tenured faculty in colleges and universities in 1994, the title emeritus was bestowed upon a retiring professor as a deserved honor. Whether older faculty members or professor emeriti are still as active as they once were, their perspective on our field and their experience can be an invaluable resource to us.

Many of these individuals have had a full career—they have risen through the ranks and achieved significant academic success. They have seen the changes that have occurred in our field and have evolved in order to be successful. They can provide significant perspective, can be invaluable in terms of how to work through institutional or political problems and can be great mentors. Furthermore they tend to have a great repertoire of amusing stories of their experience. Like the oldest storytellers, some of their anecdotes can be quite legendary.

> The great force of history comes from the fact that we carry it within us, are unconsciously controlled by it in many ways, and history is literally present in all that we do.—James Baldwin.

Key Points

- The benefits of teaching the history of urology include: (1) providing a sense of historical perspective and connection to the past (2) allow for better judgment and reasoning (3) provide a more critical approach to contemporary surgery, and (4) lead to a deeper understanding of professionalism.
- For the history of urology to be effectively taught it has to be relevant and incorporated into the regular residency schedule (taught on rounds or in the operating room, as part of introductory slides to a lecture, in a journal club setting, and in a formal dedicated lecture).
- The William P. Didusch Center for Urologic History is an excellent resource for studying the history of urology as is the annual AUA History Exhibit.
- The history of an academic institution can be used to build institutional pride and inspire its current members. Departmental newsletters can serve to further acknowledge and celebrate success, introduce new residents/faculty/staff, announce upcoming events and lectureships, keep alumni in touch with and connected to the department, help with departmental fundraising and finally chronicle the history of the department.
- Patients may also find small historical anecdotes regarding their current treatment or illness interesting and a prompt for interesting conversations.
- Emeritus Professors can serve as great mentors and provide a unique perspective on the changes in our field.

Acknowledgements Tupper Stevens for the photographs used in this chapter and for her tireless work at the William P. Didusch Center for Urologic History.

References

1. Parihar S, Kaur RJ, Singh S. Flashback and lessons learnt from history of pandemics before COVID-19. J Family Med Prim Care. 2021;10:2441–9.
2. Pan K, Goel A, Akin LR, Patel SR. Through plagues and pandemics: the evolution of medical face masks. RIMJ 2020:73–75.
3. Gawande A. Amid the coronavirus crisis, a regimen for reëntry. The New Yorker. May 13, 2020.
4. Peckham R. COVID-19 and the anti-lessons of history. Lancet. 2020;395:P850-852.
5. Patel SR, Nakada SY. Standing on the shoulders of giants: teaching the history of urology. Urology. 2013;81(6):1131–4.
6. Ojanuga D. The medical ethics of the "father of gynaecology', Dr J Marion Sims. J Med Ethics. 1993;19:28–31.
7. Gruen RL, Arya J, Cosgrove EM, et al. Professionalism in surgery. J Am Coll Surg. 2003;197:605–9.
8. Coughlin SS, Etheredge GD, Metayer C, et al. Remember Tuskegee: public health student knowledge of the ethical significance of the Tuskegee Syphilis Study. Am J Prev Med. 1996;12:242–6.
9. Osler W. A note on the teaching of the history of medicine. BMJ. 1902;2:93.

10. Miller G. The teaching of medical history in the United States and Canada: report of a field survey. Bull Hist Med. 1969;43:259–67.
11. Patel SR, Caldamone AA. Sir Denis Browne: contributions to pediatric urology. J Pediatr Urol. 2010;6:496–500.
12. Herman JR. Urology: A View Through the Retrospectroscope. Hagestown, MD: Harper & Row, Publishers Inc; ©1973.
13. Murphy LJT. The History of Urology. Charles C Thomas Publisher, Springfield IL, ©1972.
14. Landes RR, Bush RB, Zorgniotti AW. Perspectives in Urology: The Official American Urological Association History of Urology. Volume 1. AUA and Hoffman-La Roche, ©1976
15. Ballenger EG, Frontz WA, Hamer HG, Lewis B. History of Urology, Volumes 1 & 2, The Williams & Wilkins Company, Baltimore MD, ©1933
16. Moran ME. Urolithiasis: A Comprehensive History, Springer, New York, ©2014.
17. Patel SR, Moran ME, Nakada SY. The History of Technologic Advancements in Urology, Springer International Publishing AG, Switzerland, ©2018.
18. Young HH. Foreward. J Urol. 1917;1:1–2.
19. Morales P. Why this journal? 1973;1:81.
20. Patel SR. A tale of two journals: An analysis of history articles published from 1973 to 2017. IJUH. 2021;1:3–5.
21. Scott WW, William P. Didusch (1895–1981) J Urol. 1981;126:423.
22. Engel RM, The William P. Didusch Museum of the American Urological Association. J Urol. 1998;160:2450–2451.

Chapter 19
Crisis Management for Physicians

Kyle A. Richards

> "Never let a good crisis go to waste!"
>
> -Winston Churchill

What is a Crisis?

Managing a crisis is a key tenet of physician leadership. Some leaders thrive in crisis situations, whereas others struggle to rise to the occasion. But what exactly defines a crisis? For instance, one person's "crisis" might be another's average day at work. A crisis can have various levels of impact ranging from an individual (urologist), a small team (operating room), an entire organization (health system), a whole country (socialized healthcare), or the entire globe (global pandemic). A crisis as defined by Koster and Politis-Norton is "a major, abrupt and often unexpected event that has a potentially negative outcome for an organization and its employees, products, services, financial situation and reputation [1]."

An "issue" is often a prelude to a crisis and differs in the level of magnitude. If issues are identified and managed correctly, a crisis may be averted. However, it is important to note that external factors beyond your control such as media coverage, patient related factors, or health system constraints may have a huge influence on the transition from an issue to a crisis.

Crises in Urology

There are many historical examples of issues and crises outside of urology that have been well reported by mainstream media: The United States government's response to the COVID-19 pandemic; benzene contamination in Perrier water (1990) [2]; tampering of paracetamol (acetaminophen) with cyanide [Tylenol ®; Johnson & Johnson] in 1982 leading to 7 deaths in Chicago [1]; and use of performance

K. A. Richards (✉)
Department of Urology, The University of Wisconsin School of Public Health,
Madison, WI, USA
e-mail: richardsk@urology.wisc.edu

© The Author(s), under exclusive license to Springer Nature Switzerland AG 2022
S. Y. Nakada and S. R. Patel (eds.), *Navigating Organized Urology*,
https://doi.org/10.1007/978-3-031-05540-9_19

enhancing drugs in Major League Baseball. These are just a few examples of modern-day crises that required each individual or organization to manage accordingly. There are lessons to be learned in studying prior crises to help manage future issues and crises as they develop. It is not a matter of "if" but "when" the next crisis will occur. As the speed of communication has accelerated in the twenty-first century with the 24-h news cycle, organizations and individuals are potentially more susceptible to "bad" news and issues escalating into crises. Social media, conspiracy theorists, and non-traditional media outlets may also contribute to the spread of misinformation causing the crisis to have an enhancing impact on all involved parties.

Urologists are certainly not immune to crisis and should work to develop some comfort in dealing with or responding to workplace crises. Many urologists have been in the operating room under stressful situations and at some point, in their career will encounter unexpected issues that arise intra-operatively. For example, the urologist who is having issues progressing during a radical prostatectomy because the prostate is densely adherent to adjacent structures, could call a colleague to come help or continue by themselves. If the urologist decides to continue without calling their colleague and the patient sustains a large rectal injury, the issue has now become a crisis. Another example could involve an independent private practice group which is having challenges maintaining autonomy and independence as other independent medical groups are being bought out by larger managed care health systems. Finally as we have seen, the American Urological Association faced a crisis when it had to quickly pivot from an in-person annual meeting to a completely virtual platform during the COVID-19 pandemic. Each of these crises are germane to urologists and having a plan of action in mind when confronted with similar scenarios is useful to help navigate these stormy waters.

Crisis Management Strategies

The primary goal of crisis management is to limit the harm a crisis causes on stakeholders and the organization. An intra-operative complication could constitute a crisis especially if rare or unexpected. Once the event or complication has taken place, are there steps that can be taken to mitigate downstream harms? Crisis management in essence is high level problem-solving and decision making, and there have been efforts to build an evidence-based approach to identify philosophies that offer the most utility to crisis managers [3]. High level problem-solving requires leaders that are empathetic, honest, and can make wise decisions (which is easier said than done!). The decision makers need swift action and active implementation of strategic interventions to manage the crisis effectively. Lastly, it is critical to be willing to evolve as new problems and factors may emerge. Based on the best available most consistent evidence, Coombs suggested that 3 factors are most critical in crisis management (timing, victim focus, and misinformation/denial) [4].

1. *Timing*

The organization or the individual should be the first to report the crisis. The concept of timing has also been evaluated in the justice system and is known as "stealing thunder" whereby if there is a weakness in the defense's case, the defendants should raise the weakness before the prosecution has a chance to do so [5]. Greater damage is done if the prosecution raises the weakness. Similar findings have been noted in crisis communication research [6, 7]. It greatly benefits the organization or the individual to be the first to report the issue or crisis rather than stakeholders finding out through the media or second-hand. The "stealing thunder" approach seems counterintuitive, but this is where the leader needs to be transparent, honest, and timely. When the patient sustains an intra-operative complication, this is where the surgeon, as leader, should disclose what occurred immediately after the operation. Withholding these details will more likely lead to more problems for the surgeon down the road especially as patients and families have increasing immediate access to all their medical records including all operative and clinical notes.

2. *Victim focus*

All communications and messaging should be victim centric. The victim is any stakeholder that sustained actual harm (physical, psychological, and/or financial) or perceived harm. For example, the patient that sustained the complication is the victim, but their spouse may also be a victim due to psychological and/or financial harms they may incur (or even physical if the spouse passes out and bumps their head reacting to the bad news). When the response is victim focused, the victim(s) believes that the organization or individual is trying to help them and to make things right if possible. Public safety messages are critical strategies to lessen the harm a crisis might inflict and should include specific, easy to understand, details regarding the crisis with clear recommendations for stakeholders to act on to prevent additional harm from the event. An example of these challenges was seen in the United States federal response to the COVID-19 pandemic in 2020 as different government agencies and leaders were providing conflicting public safety messaging. Additionally, victims need messaging that is sympathetic, supportive (resources for counseling or support groups), and provides steps to prevent the crisis from worsening or happening again [8].

The victim-centered strategy has been shown to decrease reputational damage of the organization or individual, but sometimes empathetic messaging may have limited efficacy. If repeated crises have plagued the organization, the stakeholder may be less likely to find the organization's messaging to be credible and may perceive the organization as being careless, negligent, and/or responsible for the crisis (i.e., "that hospital has a reputation for high perioperative mortality rates"). In this scenario, it may be necessary to formulate an apology or even consider financial compensation to the victim(s). Traditionally, physicians were concerned that apologizing could create more malpractice troubles, but this rarely is the case [9]. A well thought out and sincere apology creates more trust between all parties and shows the victim that the individual or organization is human and fallible as well.

Lastly, the victim-centered messaging should be managed aggressively and not passively. An active approach will seek out all stakeholders potentially impacted by the crisis and use numerous and frequent forms of communication including media outlets, social media, emails, press conferences, etc. The messaging will be consistent and easy to understand. This may initially harm the organization's reputation, but research has shown that reputation rebounds faster from aggressive communication approaches compared to more passive approaches [10].

3. *Misinformation and Denial*

A critical crisis management component includes an aggressive educational strategy to ward off any incorrect or inaccurate information. In addition, it may be tempting for an individual or organization to deny any involvement or responsibility in the crisis, but this strategy has been shown to create a potential "double crisis." If the organization denies involvement, once all the facts (real or misinformed) emerge, the organization will have sustained more significant reputational damage and the second public relations crisis will emerge [11, 12]. A denial strategy is in complete contrast to the victim-focused strategy discussed above and should be avoided at all cost. For instance, if your patient sustains a complication during surgery, denying any involvement or responsibility as the surgeon would be counterproductive even if the responsibility may be ambiguous. Accepting responsibility does not assign blame but can create trust and open dialogue between the surgeon and key stakeholders (patient and family).

Nevertheless, denial may be an appropriate strategy when confronted with a misinformation crisis. A misinformation crisis occurs when inaccurate or untrue information is at the root cause. Misinformation crises are becoming increasingly common via social media, the internet, and non-traditional media outlets. During the COVID-19 pandemic, we have seen numerous "treatments" labeled as fact on the internet but were lacking in high quality evidence-based medicine as being effective therapies for the virus. Leaders must act quickly and aggressively in these situations to debunk the misinformation and provide counterevidence to help diffuse the situation [13, 14]. Despite best efforts by leaders to change the narrative, the damage may have already been done and key stakeholders may refuse to see things differently.

Paracrises and Social Media: The Bleeding Edge

When most surgeons think about the bleeding edge, a vivid memory surfaces of a challenging time attaining adequate hemostasis in the operating room. However, in crisis management research, the bleeding edge refers to the emergence of new problems where research evidence is lacking in providing guidance for best practice management strategies [4]. With the emergence of social media platforms over the past decade, organizations and/or individuals are at increased risk of social media crises. These are often initiated by stakeholders, have the appearance of a crisis (but are more like mini-crises or paracrises), demand a dialogue response, and are more like a form of risk management [15]. There is less robust existing evidence in how to combat these paracrises.

Organizations or individuals that engage with their stakeholder via social media need to be careful regarding the content it posts. They have a moral and social standard to adhere to and posts that fail to meet these standards could result in a paracrisis. When the organization realizes the error in judgement, swift resolution can be achieved by publicly acknowledging the mistake and promising to not make the mistake again. Unfortunately, if the organization is a repeat offender, an all-out public relations crisis may ensue and be difficult to mitigate.

As noted above, stakeholders are often the driving force behind paracrises via 3 different mechanisms:

1. Customer service
2. Venting
3. Challenge

Understanding these mechanisms will assist you in developing an effective crisis management strategy at this bleeding edge.

Customer Service: This occurs when the stakeholder makes the public aware of an issue related to the service provided by the individual or organization. For example, a patient has been sitting in the waiting room for over 1 h to see their urologist. After a lengthy wait and no explanation from the clinic staff, the patient decides to leave and posts an angry video on social media chastising the urology practice. This must be publicly addressed by the organization or else the organization risks damage to its reputation. This can also escalate to a crisis if the problem persists or if stakeholders perceive the paracrisis as one causing harm.

Venting: The main difference between customer service and venting is that the stakeholders are angry about a problem that cannot be resolved and is intended to hurt the organization. They often attack the organization using its own social medial platforms. It is best for the organization to not respond to venting even if comments may be detrimental to the organization or individual [16]. A key factor is distinguishing the difference between customer service and venting as the management strategy differs.

Challenge: When key stakeholders publicly challenge an organization's behavior or actions, their reputation is at stake and a reputational crisis may occur. These types of challenges and risks may be on the rise due to easy access to the internet and social media platforms [17]. Challenges often are related to complex potentially polarizing social issues that may or may not have a right or wrong answer including race, politics, disparities, human rights, or social injustices to name a few. Because of the complexity of these social issues, the organization may have to make a difficult decision whether to respond to the challenge and what position they should take (knowing they may not be able to please all parties). For example, nurses at your local hospital threaten to strike as they challenge the hospital for better working conditions, wages, and benefits. The organization will need to carefully craft a response to these challenges to prevent a full-blown crisis whereby the nurses go on strike, the hospital reputation takes a hit, and other stakeholders (i.e., patients) suffer as well.

Conclusions

Crises in the medical field occur with regularity and can have a wide range of impact on one's professional life. Understanding key tenets in crisis management can prepare one to navigate the journey with more success and confidence. While there may be some nuance and philosophical differences in how to approach any given crisis, the following are 6 core ideas that have emerged from the best research-based evidence [4]:

1. Release information regarding a crisis before anyone else from the outside and have an articulate spokesperson
2. Aggressively communicate information using multiple avenues including the internet
3. Immediately inform victims how to physically protect themselves if applicable
4. Immediately provide victims psychologic support (details about the event, sympathy, corrective action, and counseling) if applicable
5. Reputation recovers quicker from aggressive active communication
6. Denial strategy is only effective in combating true misinformation or rumors

In your next crisis at work, you will have the tools and preparation to lean in and accept the challenge as opposed to running in the opposite direction. Strong leaders thrive in these situations.

References

1. Koster MC, Politis-Norton H. Crisis management strategies. Drug Saf. 2004;27(8):603–8.
2. Goldberg RA. The food wars: a potential peace. J Law Med Ethics. 2000;28(4):39–45.
3. Pfeffer J, Sutton RI. Evidence-based management. Harv Bus Rev. 2006;84(1):62.
4. Coombs WT. State of crisis communication: Evidence and the bleeding edge. Res J Instit Public Relat. 2014;1(1):1–12.
5. Williams KD, Bourgeois MJ, Croyle RT. The effects of stealing thunder in criminal and civil trials. 1993;17(6):597.
6. Arpan LM, Pompper D. Stormy weather: Testing "stealing thunder" as a crisis communication strategy to improve communication flow between organizations and journalists. Public Relat Rev. 2003;29(3):291–308.
7. Claeys AS, Cauberghe V. Crisis response and crisis timing strategies, two sided of the same coin. Public Relat Rev. 2012;38(1):83–8.
8. Coombs WT. Ongoing crisis communication: Planning, managing, and responding (4th ed.) 2015. Thousand Oaks, CA: Sage.
9. Tyler L. Liability means never being able to say you're sorry corporate guild, legal constraints, and defensiveness in corporate communication. Manag Commun Q. 1997;11(1):51–73.
10. Moran R, Gregory JR. Post crisis: engage-or fly low? Brunswick Rev. 2014;8:52–4.

11. Frandsen F, Johansen W. Apologizing in a globalizing world: crisis communication and apologetic ethics. Corp Commun Int J. 2010;15(4):350–64.
12. Grebe SK. Things can get worse: How mismanagement of a crisis response strategy can cause a secondary to double crisis: the example of the AWB corporate scandal. Corporate Commun Int J. 2013;18(1):70–86.
13. DiFonzo N, Bordia P. How top PR professionals handle hearsay: corporate rumors, their effects, and strategies to manage them. Public Relat Rev. 2000;26(2):173–90.
14. Kimmel AJ, Audrain-Pontevia AF. Analysis of commercial rumors from the perspective of marketing managers: rumor prevalence, effects, and control tactics. J Market Commun. 2010;16(4):239–253.
15. Coombs WT, Holladay SJ. The paracrisis: the challenges of publicly managing crisis prevention. Public Relat Rev. 2012;38(3):408–15.
16. Gregoire Y, Laufer D, Tripp TM. A comprehensive model of customer direct and indirect revenge: understanding the effects of perceived greed and customer power. J Acad Mark Sci. 2010;38(6):738–58.
17. King BG. The tactical disruptiveness of social movements: sources of market mediated disruption in corporate boycotts. Soc Probl. 2011;58(4):491–517.

Chapter 20
Practical Lessons Learned from the Covid-19 Pandemic

Hunter Wessells

Introduction

Urologists faced a range of difficult challenges during the first weeks and months of the Covid-19 pandemic (COVID), reflecting the unknown nature of the SARS-CoV-19 pathogen and its infectivity, the rapidity with which it would impact health systems, and the additional issue of supply chain disruptions. At the outset, leaders assessed and managed risk to a number of stakeholders. These included the urology patient at various locations and types of care; surgeon, staff, and trainee safety and wellbeing; interruption of research activities; and compliance with regulations across multiple contexts and organizations [1]. As the pandemic persisted, these concerns were replaced by longer term effects including well-being of personnel and the myriad consequences of reduced clinical volume. Organizations and units that had the autonomy and flexibility to respond rapidly could adapt most successfully to the complex and changing landscape. As a counterweight to the need for adaptation during crisis, a set of core values and guiding principles proved essential for decision-making around emerging ethical and equity challenges. This chapter highlights some of the broad themes requiring significant leadership effort during COVID and the innovations and enduring new approaches coming out of this period of intense organizational disruption.

H. Wessells (✉)
Department of Urology, University of Washington School of Medicine, 1959 NE Pacific St, Box 356510, Seattle, WA 98195, United States
e-mail: wessells@uw.edu

© The Author(s), under exclusive license to Springer Nature Switzerland AG 2022
S. Y. Nakada and S. R. Patel (eds.), *Navigating Organized Urology*,
https://doi.org/10.1007/978-3-031-05540-9_20

Chain of Command

In crisis and in normal times, leaders act as integrators of information, providing situational awareness, clear communication, decision-making, and delegation along chains of command. Institutional organizational structure suits the needs of day-to-day functions; the pandemic served to clarify and reinforce the responsibilities of Service Chiefs, Vice Chairs, Program Directors, and Lab Directors in our academic department. COVID response strategy overall, surge planning, and personnel redeployment were under the direction of the Chair on the premise that determining who was deployed to the "front lines" was among the responsibilities with the greatest consequences. Operating room and ambulatory oversight and adaptations were assigned to separate Vice Chairs because the problems and solutions differed significantly. Trainees remained under the supervision of their respective Program Directors; research and administrative concerns fell to the department Director and Vice Chair of Research. Related to the chain of command was the need for a succession plan in case of illness. With no defined hierarchy below the Chair, we had to designate additional levels of responsibility.

Making sure that every individual in the department knew to whom they should look for direction was an early lesson, and reinforced the value of following these same reporting structures under normal working circumstances as well as during crisis. For our department, the assignment of pandemic work went to the team member with the skills best suited to the task, with each individual working "in their lane" as independently as possible, with the least redundancy. We anticipate that the clarity gained during COVID will allow for more efficient division of labor long term.

Communication must go up and down the chain of command to inform people and integrate information coming in from many sources. **Up-to-date organizational rosters with appropriate emergency contact information are essential**. One of the first actions we took was to make sure that we had cell phone information on all members to push text messages for urgent or emergent updates regarding call, redeployment, and vaccination roll-outs. Given the problems clinicians face in maintaining email inboxes, **we have expanded the use of coordinated text messaging to alert faculty and staff about communications that require immediate attention**.

Despite having highly reliable data on Covid transmission and modeling, course correction was frequent, and required regular recommunication and revision of plans. We co-opted an existing committee dedicated to integration of hospital, department and practice plan leaders, and converted it into twice weekly COVID meetings. As the pandemic waxed and waned, the frequency of such meetings could be dialed up or down quickly.

Personnel Deployments

Workforce issues were one of the first things to require resolution. Using the communication strategies mentioned above, we could tell people whether to stay home or go to work. This type of communication and deployment would be no different than in an earthquake, hurricane, tsunami, or other mass casualty situations. We needed to be able to have more people report to a certain location or stay away from another location, and relied on broadcasts via text messaging. Platooning of physicians into shifts was adopted at many centers; this allows appropriate numbers of trainees to be deployed given fluctuating clinical volumes. As the pandemic worsened, and staffing shortages threatened our institution's ability to maintain care across different hospital inpatient units, we transitioned to contingency staffing. Under these conditions, **we enunciated a "duty to care" as the ethical underpinning for the request that every member of the Department sign up for "COVID shifts"** [2]. Some additional subtleties of deployment were uncovered during the pandemic. Individuals on specific work visas must physically report to work in order to maintain visa eligibility. Fortunately, we were able to deploy these individuals to basic science research laboratories safely, in compliance with governmental regulations. Similarly, CMS has expectations that residents work on-site in clinics or hospitals, and thus when we platooned residents to keep a portion of them out of risk of SARS-COVID-19 infection, we needed GME sign-off in order to compliantly have residents work from home on didactics, quality improvement projects, research, or telemedicine.

Patient Care Operations

Care delivery was dramatically affected during COVID and is the subject of other chapters in this book. Triage and reduction in care in the operating room followed the Joint Statement Roadmap for Maintaining Essential Surgery created by the American College of Surgeons with several other organizations [3].

In the emergency department (ED), rapid disposition of non-Covid patients was essential to maintain ED capacity during the COVID surge. Rapid urologic evaluation and willingness to accept patients to our service prior to completion of workup was implemented. **This approach may prove valuable in reducing wait times in the ED under normal conditions and should be considered as a potential QI intervention when ongoing ED capacity issues or delays in consultant response exist.**

Within many institutions, telemedicine was the most important innovation to protect workforce, patients, and allow triage of urologic care. We were able to do this using a big bang approach for go-live, minimizing additional training. An unexpected area which required significant management was the restriction of visitation to patients to prevent the spread of Covid-19. This suspension did create significant distress for cancer patients and other acutely ill individuals and their families. Managing expectations of patients and families around visitations was essential to support front line nursing staff and principles of health equity that could be compromised by differential treatment.

Education Programs

Education programs were significantly impacted by the reduction in case volume and the need to protect workforce. The platooning described above allowed us to run residents in shifts. Only the fact that the period of greatest reduction came near the end of the academic year and only lasted two months prevented us from having significant delays in graduation. Many innovations in delivering the educational curriculum using videoconferencing were enacted during the pandemic, and a key question for leadership is when and if ever will we return to the same structure. **Institutions with very decentralized programs, many different sites of operating rooms, different OR start times, and the like, will likely see the persistence of videoconferencing over in person meetings far beyond the pandemic**.

Recruitment of trainees went surprisingly well given the fact that we only rarely used video interviewing platforms prior to Covid. The fact that these were well established in other industries was reassuring, and it is certain that **many of these interview innovations will be retained to improve the effectiveness of interviewing**. It is notable that there was a significant reduction in cost to both institutions and applicants as a result of the remote interviewing, which could be considered a factor enhancing equity, diversity, and inclusion in our recruitment processes for trainees.

Clinical Research

Clinical trial activities were significantly curtailed during Covid because human subjects and research personnel could not safely be brought into clinical environments. As institutions became comfortable with resumption of clinical care, researchers adopted a number of new strategies. These included engaging data safety monitoring boards and IRBs; reviewing trial experience and waiving requirements that would not jeopardize safety or scientific rigor; and expansion through national recruitment and developing new partnerships for remote recruiting [4]. As a result, previously precluded activities such as remote consenting and remote recruiting of research participants became acceptable [5, 6]. **These clinical trial innovations will likely persist and expand, particularly since there are no specific barriers to recruiting across state lines** as long as medical care is not being delivered.

Financial

The finances of every organization were dramatically impacted by Covid-19. Revenue, compensation, and incentives are three areas that particularly impacted clinical departments. As shown in Fig. 20.1, the productivity of the Department of Urology in its adult urology activities was reduced significantly during the first months of the pandemic. As can be seen in the Figure, the majority of this was experienced in April, with portions of March and May. It was necessary to use reserve funds to cover expenses during this interval, because revenue based on clinical activity was substantially reduced. The reduction equaled approximately one month's revenue. Health systems suffered massive reductions in volume and revenue and had similar constraints. Hospitals and practice plans separately tapped into government relief funds. Our hospitals used these funds to support staff FTE generally and to maintain payment for physician services. The amount of relief that went separately to practice plans depended on the relationship of the two entities within a given health system. Private practices and large group practices unaffiliated with hospitals received larger direct payments.

A number of belt tightening measures were implemented. **Our department took the approach that the most vulnerable individuals in our salary structure, including classified and professional staff who are not physicians, should not bear the burden of immediate expense reduction.** Expense reduction tools implemented included reduction of compensation for senior leadership; limiting new recruitments to positions of critical importance; postponement of capital expenses which were not mission critical; voluntary furloughs for professional and classified staff; faculty leave of absence; deferred maintenance of facilities; and as a

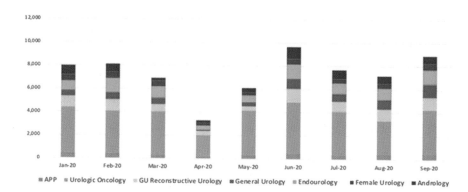

Fig. 20.1 Clinical Productivity Reduction (in wRVUs) and Recovery during initial phases of the COVID-19 Pandemic. Note dramatic reduction in April 2020, the differential impact on subspecialties (pediatric urology data not included), and the recovery in June and subsequent months. From Sekar RR, Holt SK, Meno J, McKenzie R, Wessells H: Urologic Emergency Care in the COVID-19 Pandemic Era. In Wessells H, Horie S, Gomez RG Eds. *Clinical Guide to Urological Emergencies*. Wiley, Oxford, 2021 with permission

last resort layoffs of professional and classified staff. The simplest reduction approach was restriction on travel which, while a small component of most budgets overall, nevertheless was easy to implement. **Overall, these measures were successful in reducing expenses, and serve as a model for managing future variation in revenue due to disruptions such as recession, contracting failures, and other disasters.**

Compensation to faculty physicians and trainees at our institution was not reduced at the base salary level. Notably, some institutions reduced expenses by cutting base salary and/or retirement benefits [7], the latter causing some of the greatest long-term impact on the recipients of those benefits because of the loss of compounded growth of retirement benefits.

Incentive payments, which are distributed quarterly or semi-annually in our practice plan, were an obvious mechanism to adjust compensation to urologists in parallel with the reduction in wRVU and revenue. **The principles of equity and protection, which were used to consider staff cuts, were also taken into consideration when determining how to manage physician incentives, which make up 15–25% of the compensation of faculty in the practice plan.**

Incentive payments throughout the COVID pandemic have represented a particular challenge because access to the operating rooms and triage of essential cases varied significantly across departments and units within departments. Urology practices are largely elective, with a variable portion of surgical cases, such as obstructive stones and cancers, that are considered of immediate urgency. This created differential access to the operating room and patient volume such that some faculty members could continue to work at near normal levels while others were at a much reduced rate (see Fig. 20.1). While our incentive plan traditionally allocates the majority of the incentive based on individual work relative value units (wRVU), we created COVID contingencies whereby incentives were split such that the incentive pool would be distributed via a mix of wRVUs and clinical FTE (cFTE) assignment. Under this scenario, an individual with a large clinical FTE who could not perform as much surgery due to triage and cancellation of elective cases, yet still was working in clinic, would see a mitigation in the impact of reduced wRVU on their compensation. The variation in access to patients and OR capacity has persisted throughout successive waves of COVID, and thus **we have modified our incentive plan to allocate the distribution according to a mix of wRVU and cFTE that can be varied according to events and mitigate fluctuations in surgeon access to patients, OR capacity, and other factors affecting clinical productivity.**

Perspectives

The COVID-19 pandemic required leaders to make decisions without precedent, and without time to seek input that would be obtained under usual conditions. Having a defined set of core values that could serve as reference and guidance was an important resource. Communicating our intentions and enunciating values associated with a decision was more important than almost any single decision.

Engaging our most important reserves, namely the human commitment and resiliency within our people, was arguably a leaders' highest priority. Safeguards for staff on the front line revolved around personal protective equipment and testing; for students and residents, educational needs had to be balanced. As the pandemic worsened, and staffing shortages threatened our institution's ability to maintain care across different hospital inpatient settings, we transitioned to contingency staffing. Under these conditions, we invoked the "duty to care" as the ethical basis for asking every member of the department to sign up for "COVID shifts." We expanded the factors used to make decisions about compensation, and paid particular attention to disparities created by unequal access to resources, based on rank, location, job title, and subspecialty. Our institutional Health Equity Blueprint was key to managing families seeking visitation rights, ensuring applicants access to our training programs, and guiding triage of cases for deferred care.

Adaptability and flexibility proved invaluable in the face of the pandemic and the complexity of the disruption. As a department that has always placed an emphasis on innovation and responding to opportunities, these traits were ingrained and could be repurposed to respond to crisis. The longer term challenge is more daunting: how do we ask people to do more, contribute to financial recovery, and work with less with no end in sight? The sacrifices and efforts made to date will seem even more meaningful if we re-envision the future of Urology in terms of permanent changes to the status quo. Making sure we use this moment of opportunity to break out of entrenchment and recreate, reinvent the future will require that we leverage agreement of interests using specific methods as part of leadership repertoire. Leaders will need to ask strategic questions, as we collectively reflect on how we got to the previous status quo. Leadership in crisis can engage the next generation of leaders within our institutions to solve previously insolvable problems.

References

1. Society of Academic Urologists. SAU Chairs' roundtable Webinar: sharing experiences to cope with the COVID-19 pandemic. https://sauweb.org/resources/covid-19-resources.aspx. Accessed 25 Oct 2020.
2. Dudzinski DM, Hoisington BY, Brown CE. Ethics lessons from Seattle's early experience with COVID-19. Am J Bioeth. 2020;20(7):67–74.
3. American College of Surgeons. COVID-19: Guidance for Triage of Non-Emergent Surgical Procedures. https://www.facs.org/covid-19/clinical-guidance/triage.
4. Urinary Stone Disease Research Network (USDRN) Investigators. Impact of COVID-19 on Prevention of Urinary Stones with Hydration (PUSH) study: challenges and opportunities for future trials. J Urol. 2021;206(3):502–504.
5. FDA guidance on conduct of clinical trials of medical products during COVID-19 public health emergency: guidance for industry, investigators, and institutional review boards. Updated June 3, 2020. https://www.fda.gov/media/136238/download. Accessed 23 Apr 2020.

6. Mitchell EJ, Ahmed K, Breeman S, et al. It is unprecedented: trial management during the COVID-19 pandemic and beyond. Trials. 2020;21:784.
7. https://hub.jhu.edu/2020/04/21/jhu-prepares-for-financial-challenges-from-covid-19/.

Chapter 21
Re-Evaluating Yourself

Stephen Y. Nakada

Now that we have arrived at the end of the journey of "Navigating Organized Urology," a re-evaluation discussion is in order. Chapter 1, "Knowing Yourself," focused on the here and now; but we will now focus on key attributes to moving forward once you have experience in the roles of all of the prior chapters. Probably the clearest truth to most people in re-evaluation is, while your core values and styles do not really change, the details, impressions you make, and the way you present yourself does. In my opinion, it is the external factors, that we typically do not control, that lead much of the way forward. That is not to say you do not control your future, but more to say a career is typically about a series of decisions you make based on your opportunities and timing. The overall strategy does not change; performance first, purpose second, and passion if possible. At this stage, some straightforward, yet important questions to ask yourself are, "How am I different today than when I first started?", and "What has worked well?", "Have I enjoyed the ride thus far?". Harder questions include, "Have I made any key mistakes, and what have I learned from them?", "Am I truly on the course that I want to be on?", "What remains as areas of improvement for me?" (Fig. 21.1) This chapter will address these questions and potential answers, and how those answers will shape the way forward.

A. Setting future goals

First off, if you are reading this book you likely have some future remaining, or in other words, "you still have some runway." While I think setting your first set of goals (Chap. 1) is important, undoubtedly the next set of goals, or your true "long term vision statement" has become more pressing if not done so already. This is because you have some performance history, and your window for opportunity is

S. Y. Nakada (✉)
Department of Urology, UWMF Practice Plan, UW Medical Foundation Centennial Building, 1685 highland Avenue, Madison, WI 53705-2281, USA
e-mail: nakada@urology.wisc.edu

Easy questions to ask yourself

"How am my different today than when I first started?"

"What has worked well?'

"Have I enjoyed the ride so far?"

Hard questions to ask yourself:

"Have I made any key mistakes, and what have I learned from them?"

"Am I truly on the course that I want to be on?"

"What remains as areas of improvement for me?"

Fig. 21.1 Easy Questions to Ask Yourself

smaller, and most likely you have changed, probably for the better. When setting goals, to understand how you've changed is important, as your value system and strategy can become more focused. As you progress in your career, the idea of focusing on just performance, and everything else will take care of itself, begins to lose value. By now, you have some idea if you are leaning towards research, innovation, leadership, education, or industry. That said, available opportunities and the current trends in the field become very relevant to you, and your engagement in these trends creates much of your value. Looking at second jobs or new opportunities makes great sense, even if you do not move. In many cases, you will learn you have it best at your current job.

A substantial expense and sweat equity has been put into your career by both you and your home department or group at this stage, so any opportunity will have to really add value to your career or personal life. Sometimes if things aren't working out, such as your department or leadership is in transition or turmoil, there is a sudden need for change, and that can be the best thing to do. One important question is, who can advise you on these matters? Generally, I would be very cautious about this, and I recommend confiding in a trusted, senior mentor. While your colleagues may be trustworthy, they may learn from you about an opportunity for themselves! Moreover, inevitably word gets out about either your dissatisfaction or desire to move, and this generally has negative effects on local relationships. Subordinates offer less help, and information shared at this level can be even more destabilizing.

I have spent my professional career at one institution, and cannot give personal anecdotes on the effect of changing departments, or paths. My observation is the better your performance, the more options you have. Overall, staying power has great value, although there is a cost. Changing jobs allows you to bring a new culture to the team, and you will learn much from a different system. In addition, there may just not be the opportunity you seek at your current location, necessitating the strategic move.

Personal reasons can also be powerful motivators for a midcareer move. The old adage is that it costs you 6 months of productivity to catch up from a move, but this is strictly research driven. If you need a change of environment, your productivity in fact could increase dramatically with a change of scenery. Personal moves can have the additive benefit of a more stable home environment, which can be key to success. I would always make a list of why you want to move, and why the new destination is better than your current spot. Reading both, these lists must be integrated, and relatively long for you to jump in. (Fig. 21.2).

It is at this time new goals can be set. Perhaps leadership, innovation, or educational roles are in the future. Notably, research is a tough "new" goal due to the early commitment needed to succeed. Your mentors, and Chair or Dean can be strong sounding boards. My view, based on careful observation, is that you can identify new directions that can suit you. I think the mistake many make is not to verbalize these interests at the right levels (people in this role, perhaps even not at your institution). Getting to these goals will be addressed in the next section. Regardless, your goals should be stretch goals, as most successful determined people accomplish the most using stretch goals. For instance, a goal may be to become "head of a research program" but a stretch goal may be to "become Dean".

Just a word on the "lateral transfer." Some believe this is a dangerous thing, mostly because without an inherent "win" upon arrival, your upside may be tapped out professionally early in transition. Generally, harder work will be needed to get to the next level (if that is what you seek) if you take a lateral move, as you will have to prove yourself, since the institution or group wouldn't grant you the position up front. However, your "ceiling" may be exceeded at your current institution, taking this option sometimes is the best one. There can be a sense of bitterness, or disengagement when you make a lateral transfer. This could come from further negotiation with your current leadership and colleagues, and due to a

Why do I want to move?

No more upward mobility.

Declining leadership.

Internal conflict with colleagues.

High cost of living.

Key colleagues are retiring or leaving.

Why is the new job better?

Can move into a better position immediately (not a lateral transfer).

Leadership is new, seems enlightened.

New colleagues seem engaging.

Lower cost of living.

Perfect opportunity for collaboration.

Fig. 21.2 Why Do I Want to Move?

lack of a clear understanding of your path ahead. While taking a new job may feel like a "leap of faith," even in the case of a lateral transfer, this may be the cogent decision, just try and have clarity when you can.

B. Continued personal and professional growth

There is no more powerful learning tool than close observation of high performing people, or people you hope to emulate. I jump at opportunities to work with our system leadership, first to help the cause as it is my job, but I also know I will get the added benefit of observing the leadership closely, seeing how they formulate a plan, strategy for that plan, and watch the subsequent execution. Of course, things don't always work out, which is also a learning opportunity. Similarly, with experience, I have learned to involve my faculty more in strategy and execution, both to seek their assistance and their own education.

I remember a wise chief resident once told me when I was an intern on trauma call, "the more senior I've become, the more I ask questions. So do you really expect to not have to call me tonight?" That is a powerful statement, with multiple messages: 1. I expect excellent care from us tonight, 2. Call me, not the attending, 3. I recognize your inexperience and it's okay. The astute resident can learn this valuable communication lesson, which potentially helps the resident learn how to message triage nursing, medical students and others in the emergency room. Good or bad, stressful or gleeful, there is always a learning opportunity. That's a key thing to remember.

A common question is how hard should you push your own agenda? Let's say you are an associate professor, and have not had the opportunities of others with similar abilities, backgrounds and accomplishments. Do you push this with your chair, or others, or remain silent? The first question is, are you really equivalent? Have you looked in the mirror closely enough? Your CV may look the same, but is your punctuality, reliability, and attitude equivalent? Nobody likes a nitpicker, or a complainer. I recommend rather than pushing for opportunities, I would ask about how you can help, and what you could do better. You will generally get to the same end but with more grace and aplomb than pushing your agenda. Academic urology is not always fair, but it is more transparent than many professions. In our department we have developed an internal code (Fig. 21.3). This code has multiple messages, and the list is long enough that there is something for everyone. Reading into our code, we say a few key things: be prepared, do it right, and trust the system. Next the code addresses how to behave to get back on course if the wheels come off. But they are just words, what is really accomplished here? I believe it is always good to clarify department values, as it helps each team member to work under a credo and function with less fear, as long as the values are protected. Perhaps you or your team needs a code, and perhaps it could read like this one. More importantly, start with common guidelines for behavior whenever possible. This is a case where guidelines can be more freeing than "restricting."

Ongoing development can be vital, and helpful, but pursing this in a busy time in your career is challenging. My viewpoint, as you become more senior and more skilled, is that you can buy time, and take courses or take a personal or group retreat

Fig. 21.3 House Rules

House Rules

Be yourself.

Be accountable.

Read about it first.

Delegate with discretion.

Trust that it is a meritocracy.

Rather than argue, offer suggestions.

Rather than complain, propose solutions.

to recharge. Most of us do not do this enough, and this can be very helpful. Time is the most precious commodity we have, and generally urologists do not lack for salary, unless other circumstances more personal than professional have intervened.

C. Mentorship

Mentorship is vital to most all career paths. At the beginning, you depend on it, and I hope you select well. As your momentum mounts, people will seek you out as a mentor and colleague. This is a very positive sign, and more importantly as those you mentor begin to succeed, more people will become engaged. I have learned it is best to provide authentic, clear feedback, just as you desired from your mentor.(3) Perhaps if something is outside your area of knowledge, it is most transparent to just say that, and best if you can recommend a different content expert. Once in your area of expertise, positive feedback is usually best, rather than "I wouldn't try that approach," a better answer might be "have you considered…" Regardless, when mentoring, listen carefully. There is much said in few words in these conversations. Also, be parsimonious with your comments, as they are also critically important, every word, even a sigh.

My belief is the value of both sides of the mentor–mentee relationship is substantive, and the more of these you have, the better. Someone you have mentored well will be quick to repay the favor if you need them later. In this manner, many leaders have established their "board." When something good happens, you call a board member, or all of them. When you need advice, you check your board for the best advisee to contact. Your board may include several family members and friends, perhaps an old college roommate, as well as urologists [1].

D. The Only Constant is Change- Adapting to change

This is the most important lesson in this chapter. We have addressed the various generational gaps and gender sensitivities in earlier chapters, and from all this the one thing that is clear is that the ability to change is a "superpower."

There is nothing more difficult than to change [2]. I am always wary of someone who says they are old school. To me, old school is dead school. So if you are "a little old school," you are at the very least, "a little flawed, or in the process of extinction." Old school values, such as hard work, blind passion, intense loyalty, may sound good but are far from modern or as relevant as in the past. To me, the old school approach is like riding on a horse with a rifle into battle against a fully engaged tank division. It has some charm, but the only other saving grace is that you will die painlessly and quickly.

Ego and respect are also problematic values. No matter who you are, leave your ego at the door whenever possible. If you feel the need to say or do something egotistical, leave. Do not pursue that situation in the present, and by all means do not send an angry email! Regroup, and fight another day if needed. Generally 24 h, if you have it, is the best first strategy. Reassess in your mind what happened, and decide if you in fact have a case, and if so, manage the situation with surgical precision, like resecting a cancer. If not, good for you that you walked away.

Respect is more complicated. I also worry if someone tells me they want more respect. Why? Because they are a Professor, or Section Chief, or Department Chair? Today we live in a "what have you done for me lately society," or more accurately what have you done for me today environment. You can seek respect, but in the end you earn respect, most likely every day, every hour. We work in a hierarchical environment, of rank, or full partner status in the practice setting. While important at many levels, the "privileges of membership" can be the source of serious indiscretions. Again, the emphasis must be on self-improvement, moving forward, and adapting, not living on past accomplishments and times. One of my colleagues reprimanded a young resident for addressing him by Dr. X, rather than Professor X. This got back to me, and Professor X said he had earned that title, and deserved respect. While there is some truth to that, I had trouble not visualizing him on a horse with a rifle.

So how do you learn to adapt? I have a few thoughts. Knowing yourself is really key here, as you may think you're adapting, but you're not. Ask others, watch others, and mentor others with interest. With time, you can learn a lot from your mentees, how they respond to compliments and criticism. In general, the more positive you can be the better. In social situations, your adaptive ability will show. Who is drawn to you, who asks you for advice? This can be telling. Do subordinates primarily "just pay homage" or do they appear to be interested in talking to you? What about your younger colleagues? In the end, continue to refine your approach to best meet the needs of your team [3].

Next, assume anything is possible. If someone brings an idea to you, the worst thing you can do is just shoot it down. It gives you the image of old school; any innovator would tell you that. Ironically, some of the most ridiculous statements have become the future of our field. To me, the most memorable in my era of training was the fact that "minimally invasive (laparoscopic) radical prostatectomy is dead." Then came the robot, leading Professor Mani Menon straight to every accolade organized urology can offer [4].

Finally, adaptation requires study. We covered social media in Chap. 16. This is yet another medium that some embrace and some do not. Regardless, in my view it is a critical avenue of communication and learning, but there are precautions. Those who can adapt are the "ultimate students," who keep getting better against odds. For instance, Bernhard Langer, who is over 60 years of age, is technically a better golfer than in 1985 when he won his first Masters [3]. Now urology isn't golf, but certainly history would have told Bernhard his skills would begin deteriorating after age 57, but he did not believe that [5]. We are in the process of "retiring" surgeons at 70, but *maybe*, there are some surgeons at 70 who are better than surgeons who are 45. Perhaps the young generation may have to adapt to the older generation as well.

To summarize, all of my comments in Chap. 1 and this chapter are my opinion, not fact or literature based in the practical sense. The goal of Navigating Organized Urology is to provide you with a comprehensive framework to have a successful and fulfilling career, and to this end we have called on key people that we think have exceled in their given chapter topics. I honestly have interest in your feedback, as undoubtedly, many of you in reading this will disagree, or provide valuable suggestions. Please do so, and good luck!

Key Points

1. Your career cannot be scripted, but study many scripts!
2. Education, and more importantly learning, is important at every stage. You do this EVERY day.
3. Adaptation requires leaving any old school ideals, ego, and history at the door. Change is a superpower worth mastering.
4. Embrace mentees, as well as mentors. These are lifelong relationships.
5. Create your own "board," and call on them when needed.

References

1. Michael Breed, personal communication
2. Johnson S. Who moved my cheese? 1998, G. Putnam and Sons
3. Operate with Zen, Leadership Podcast https://podcasts.apple.com/us/podcast/22-mindful-leadership-with-dr-stephen-nakada/id1579495428?i=1000540432603
4. https://www.auanet.org/about-us/aua-governance/awards/award-winners/previous-honorees
5. http://www.espn.com/golf/player/_/id/261/bernhard-langer